TRAUMATIC DENTAL INJURIES
– A Manual

Second Edition

J.O. ANDREASEN

F.M. ANDREASEN

L.K. BAKLAND

M.T. FLORES

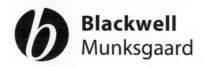
Blackwell
Munksgaard

© 2003 by Blackwell Munksgaard, a Blackwell Publishing company

Editorial Offices:
Blackwell Publishing Ltd, 9600 Garsington Road, Oxford OX4 2DQ, UK
    Tel: +44 (0)1865 776868
Blackwell Publishing Professional, 2121 State Avenue, Ames, Iowa 50014-8300, USA
    Tel: +1 515 292 0140
Blackwell Publishing Asia Pty Ltd, 550 Swanston Street, Carlton, Victoria 3053, Australia
    Tel: +61 (0)3 8359 1011

First edition published 2000
Second edition published by Blackwell Munksgaard 2003
5   2006

Library of Congress Cataloging-in-Publication Data is available

ISBN-10: 1-4051-1108-9
ISBN-13: 978-14051-1108-9

A catalogue record for this title is available from the British Library

Artwork by Henning Dalhoff Aps
Typeset in 9/12pt Helvetica and produced by
Gray Publishing, Tunbridge Wells, Kent
Printed and bound in Denmark
by Narayana Press, Odder, Denmark.

The publisher's policy is to use permanent paper from mills that operate a sustainable forestry policy, and which has been manufactured from pulp processed using acid-free and elementary chlorine-free practices. Furthermore, the publisher ensures that the text paper and cover board used have met acceptable environmental accreditation standards.

For further information on Blackwell Munksgaard, visit our website:
www.dentistry.blackwellmunksgaard.com

Preface

In this second edition, the epidemiological section on global trauma frequencies has been updated and all chapters have been revised, especially with respect to the urgency of acute treatment. Furthermore, the chapter on prevention of oral injuries has been expanded. New chapters include diagnosis of pulp and periodontal healing complications, long-term prognosis of the various trauma entities, information to the patient subsequent to emergency treatment. Finally, a chapter has been included which deals with the principles of endodontic treatment of traumatized teeth.

J. O. Andreasen, F. M. Andreasen,
L. K. Bakland, M. T. Flores
Copenhagen, January 2003

Preface to the first edition

In *Traumatic Dental Injuries – A Manual*, we present the highlights of dental traumatology in a format, which will be a ready reference for general practitioners and aid dental students in their studies. Each chapter is designed to describe the principles in the diagnosis and treatment of the specific traumatic dental injury, including treatment objectives, treatment parameters and long-term expectations based on existing long-term studies of various trauma entities. In order to standardize diagnostic and treatment procedures, examination forms and follow-up protocol are provided in the appendices. As no type of dental trauma is "perfect", a given injury type has been generated electronically by a medical artist, in order to enhance similarities and differences between the various injury groups. Periodontal and pulpal healing for the given injuries are based on recent long-term follow-up studies.

Finally, information to the public is also presented. As the best treatment result follows prompt emergency care, informed individuals at the scene of the injury can aid the dental practitioner in optimizing treatment and hopefully in preventing injuries.

It is the authors' hope that *Traumatic Dental Injuries – A Manual* will fill the gap in dental education and give dental trauma its full birthright.

J. O. Andreasen, F. M. Andreasen,
L. K. Bakland, M. T. Flores
Copenhagen, January 1999

Contributors

JENS O. ANDREASEN, DDS, ODONT DR. HC, FRCS
Department of Oral and Maxillofacial Surgery
University Hospital (Rigshospitalet)
Copenhagen
Denmark

FRANCES M. ANDREASEN, DDS, DR. ODONT
Research associate
Department of Oral and Maxillofacial Surgery
University Hospital (Rigshospitalet)
Copenhagen
Denmark

LEIF K. BAKLAND, DDS
Diplomate, American Board of Endodontics
Professor and Chairman
Department of Endodontics
Associate Dean, Advanced Education
School of Dentistry, Loma Linda University
Loma Linda, California
USA

MARIA T. FLORES, DDS
Professor of Pediatric Dentistry
Graduate Dental Faculty
University of Valparaiso
Valparaiso
Chile

Contents

Epidemiology of Traumatic Dental Injuries

OBJECTIVES **1** Recognize trauma frequencies in the primary and permanent dentitions.
2 Recognize peak incidences of trauma in relation to age.
3 Recognize typical causes of trauma.

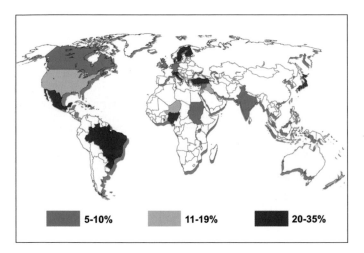

TRAUMA FREQUENCIES

The frequency of traumatic dental injuries has been examined in many countries, usually with very high figures as the result.[1-12] However, it should be considered that most of these studies represent frequencies in varying age groups, whereby these frequencies cannot be compared. When frequencies are broken down for 5- and 12-year-olds, the figures are as in the maps below.

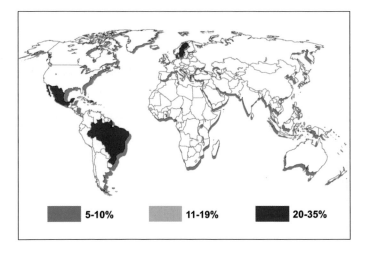

TRAUMA FREQUENCIES IN 5-YEAR-OLD CHILDREN

In 5-year-old children, approximately one-third have suffered a traumatic dental injury involving primary teeth, most often tooth luxation; and boys slightly more often than girls.[1-12]

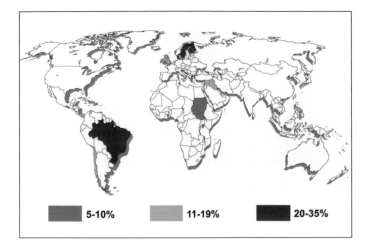

TRAUMA FREQUENCIES IN 12-YEAR-OLD CHILDREN

In 12-year-old children, 20–30% have suffered dental injuries, boys being approximately one-third more frequently affected. The typical injury is uncomplicated crown fracture.[1-12]

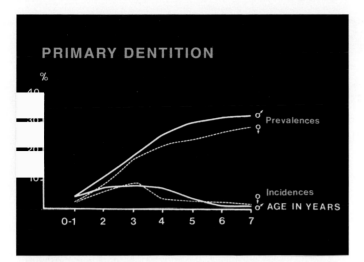

TRAUMA INCIDENCES IN THE PRIMARY DENTITION

Annual trauma incidences (i.e. the number of new injuries suffered during a year), peak incidences in the primary dentition are found at 2–3 years of age, where motor coordination is developing and the children start moving around on their own.[1-12]

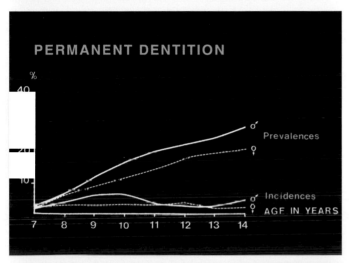

TRAUMA INCIDENCES IN THE PERMANENT DENTITION

In the permanent dentition, peak incidences for boys are found at 9–10 years, where vigorous playing and sports activities become more frequent.[1-12]

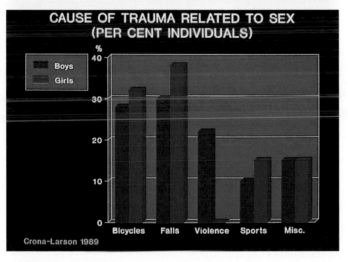

ETIOLOGY OF TRAUMA

The most common injuries in the permanent dentition are due to falls, followed by traffic injuries, acts of violence and sports.[1-13]

NOTES

_____

_____

_____

_____

_____

_____

Nature and Consequences of Trauma

OBJECTIVES
1 Describe the nature and effect of trauma.
2 Describe healing events after simple (separation) injuries to the pulp and periodontium.
3 Describe healing events after complicated (crushing) injuries to the pulp and periodontium.

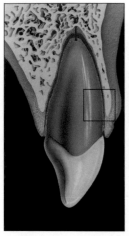

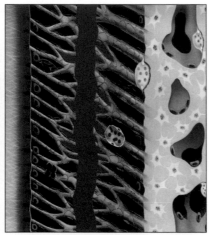

NATURE OF TRAUMA: SEPARATION INJURY

A traumatic dental injury represents acute transmission of energy to the tooth and supporting structures, which results in fracture and/or displacement of the tooth and/or separation or crushing of the supporting tissues (gingiva and bone).[14,15] In cases of separation injury (e.g. extrusive luxation), the major part of the injury consists of cleavage of intercellular structures (collagen and intercellular substance), while there is limited damage to the cells in the area of trauma. This implies that wound healing can arise from existing cellular systems with a minimum of delay.

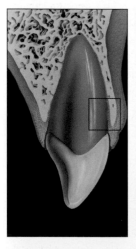

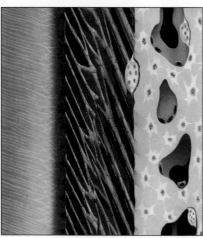

NATURE OF TRAUMA: CRUSHING INJURY

In contrast, in a crushing injury (e.g. intrusive luxation), there is extensive damage to both cellular and intercellular systems; and damaged tissue must be removed by macrophages and/or osteoclasts before the traumatized tissue can be restored. Such damage adds several weeks to the healing process and is reflected in the splinting period.

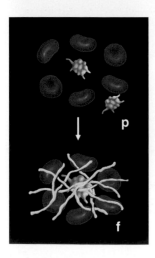

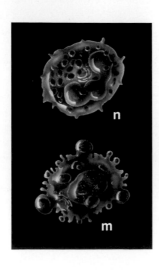

EARLY WOUND HEALING EVENTS

The immediate events following trauma include bleeding from ruptured vessels followed by coagulation.[14] The platelets (p) in the coagulum play a significant role, not only in transformation of fibrinogen to fibrin (f), but also due to their content of growth factors (e.g. platelet-derived growth factor (PGDF), transforming growth factor (TGF)-β), which initiate the wound healing process. Thereafter, an influx of neutrophilic leukocytes (n) and macrophages (m) takes place. The first cell type is concerned with infection, the second with cleaning up the area of damaged tissue and foreign bodies, assisting the neutrophilic leukocytes in defending against or combating microbial colonization, and finally in taking over the platelets' role in directing wound healing events.[14]

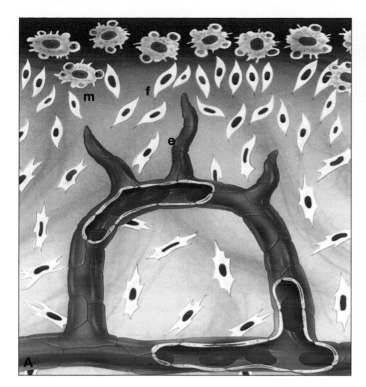

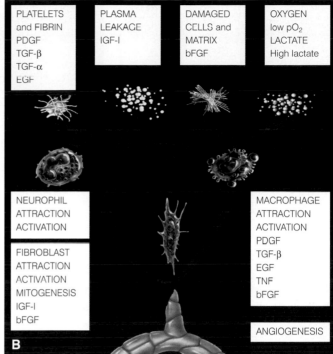

| PLATELETS and FIBRIN PDGF TGF-β TGF-α EGF | PLASMA LEAKAGE IGF-I | DAMAGED CELLS and MATRIX bFGF | OXYGEN low pO₂ LACTATE High lactate |

NEUROPHIL ATTRACTION ACTIVATION

FIBROBLAST ATTRACTION ACTIVATION MITOGENESIS IGF-I bFGF

MACROPHAGE ATTRACTION ACTIVATION PDGF TGF-β EGF TNF bFGF

ANGIOGENESIS

LATER WOUND HEALING EVENTS

Wound healing events comprise revascularization of ischemic tissue and formation of new tissue in case of tissue loss (A). In both instances, wound healing takes place by a coordinated movement of cells into the traumatized area, where macrophages (m) form the healing front, followed by endothelial cells (e) and fibroblasts (f). Vascular loops are formed in a stroma of tissue dominated by immature collagen (Type III) and proliferating fibroblasts. These cells are synchronized via chemical signals released by the involved cells and the surrounding tissue.[14] This phenomenon has been termed the wound healing module (B). This process appears to advance in the pulp and periodontium with a speed of approximately 0.5 mm a day.[1b]

Below, wound-healing responses will be described as they appear in cases of simple luxation injuries, with only separation injuries of the periodontal ligament (PDL) and the pulp, and complicated luxation injuries with crushing injuries.[15]

The few experiments carried out on simple luxation injuries indicate the following about the type and chronology of healing:

PDL: after 1 week, new collagen formation starts to unite the severed PDL fibers and results in initial consolidation of a luxated or a replanted tooth. After 2 weeks, repair of the principal fibers is so advanced that approximately two-thirds of the mechanical strength of the PDL has been regained.[15]

Pulp: in luxated teeth with a severed vascular supply, ingrowth of new vessels into the pulp starts 4 days after injury and proceeds with a speed of approximately 0.5 mm per day in teeth with open apices. Revascularization is markedly influenced by the size of the pulpo-periodontal interface, being complete and predictable in teeth with open apices (≥ 1.0 mm), and rare in teeth with a narrow apical foramen (<0.5 mm).[36]

The most significant factor that can arrest the revascularization process appears to be colonization of bacteria in the ischemic pulp tissue. The origin of these bacteria can be invasion from dentinal tubules via a crown fracture, or invasion along the blood clot in a severed PDL. Finally, bacteria can be carried to the area via the blood stream (anachoresis). Thus, it has been found that the revascularization process with its endothelial sprouts is often incontinent, allowing corpuscular elements, like erythrocytes and bacteria, to leave the blood stream.

In **complicated luxation injuries**, with **crushing or other damage of the PDL** (e.g. desiccation after avulsion), complicating sequelae may occur which result in root resorption.[16–26] These processes occur due to the loss of the protecting cementoblast layer and the epithelial rests of Mallassez along the root surface, caused by the traumatic events. When these cell layers disappear, there is free access of osteoclasts and macrophages to remove damaged PDL and cementum on the root surface.

Further events are subsequently determined by three factors:

- eventual exposure of dentinal tubules

- content of the pulp, whether ischemic and sterile or necrotic and infected

- presence of adjacent vital cementoblasts.

The combination of these factors may lead to the healing complications shown on the following pages as the wound healing module approaches the injury site.[15–18]

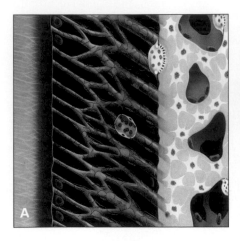
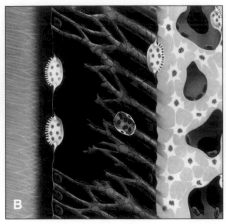
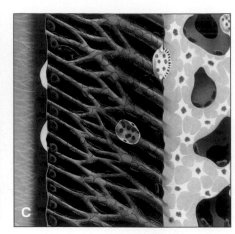

SURFACE (NONINFECTIOUS) RESORPTION

In cases of damage to the layer of the PDL closest to cementum (A), the site will be resorbed by macrophages and osteoclasts, resulting in a saucer-shaped cavity on the root surface (B). If this cavity is not in contact with dentinal tubules and the adjacent cementoblast layer is intact, this resorption cavity is repaired by new cementum and insertion of new Sharpey's fibers (C). The ligament width is normal and follows the contours of the defect.

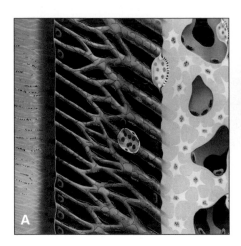
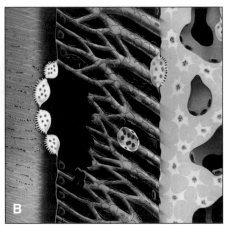
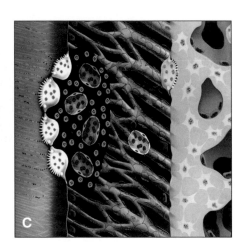

INFLAMMATORY (INFECTIOUS) RESORPTION

In the event that the initial resorption has penetrated cementum and exposed dentinal tubules, toxins from bacteria present in the dentinal tubules and/or the infected root canal can be diffused via the exposed tubules to the PDL. This results in continuation of the osteoclastic process and an associated inflammation in the PDL leading to resorption of the lamina dura and adjacent bone (B). This process is usually progressive until the root canal is exposed. If bacteria are eliminated from the root canal and/or dentinal tubules by proper endodontic therapy, the resorptive process will be arrested. The resorption cavity will then be filled in with cementum or bone, according to the type of vital tissue found next to the resorption site (PDL or bone marrow-derived tissue).

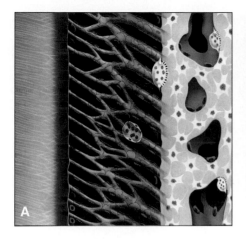
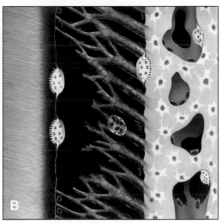
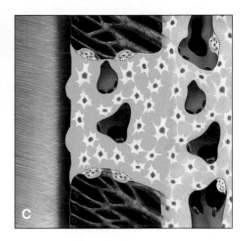

REPLACEMENT RESORPTION (ANKYLOSIS)

In cases of extensive damage to the innermost layer of the PDL, competitive healing events will take place whereby healing from the socket wall (creating bone via bone marrow-derived cells) and healing from adjacent PDL next to the root surface (creating cementum and Sharpey's fibers) will take place simultaneously.[15–19]

With cases of moderately sized injuries (1–4 mm^2), an initial ankylosis is formed (A–C). This can later be replaced with new cementum and PDL, if allowed functional mobility by the use of a semi-rigid splint, or no splinting (transient ankylosis).

With larger injuries (>4 mm^2) a transient or progressive ankylosis is created. This implies that the tooth becomes an integral part of the bone remodeling system. The entire process includes osteoclastic resorption dependent on bone remodeling processes, parathyroid hormone-induced resorption, remodeling due to function and resorption due to bacteria present in the gingival area and/or the root canal. All of these processes are very active in children and lead to gradual infraocclusion and arrested development of the alveolar process. In children, this combination of resorption processes leads to loss of ankylosed teeth within 1–5 years. In older individuals, replacement resorption is significantly slower and often allows the tooth to function for longer periods of time (i.e. 5–20 years).

TRANSIENT MARGINAL BREAKDOWN AND TRANSIENT APICAL BREAKDOWN OF BONE

In instances where compression of the PDL has occurred (e.g. lateral luxation and intrusion), macrophage/osteoclast removal of traumatized tissue before periodontal healing takes place, may result in a transient marginal breakdown, which is manifested by formation of gingival granulation tissue at the site of compression and a transient radiographic breakdown of the lamina dura at the site involved. After 2–3 months the periodontium will usually be rebuilt.[3] Likewise, in the apical region a transient apical breakdown may occur in teeth with closed apices in cases where pulp healing takes place after luxation injuries (i.e. extrusion, lateral luxation). In these instances a transient radiographic radiolucency is seen as a response to ingrowth of new tissue into the pulp canal.[104]

INFLUENCE OF TREATMENT ON WOUND HEALING AFTER LUXATION AND REPLANTATION AFTER AVULSION

The value of treatment procedures, such as repositioning and splinting, has not yet been adequately investigated. Evidence to date demonstrates the following (see pages 14 and 15).

NOTES

_____

_____

_____

_____

_____

_____

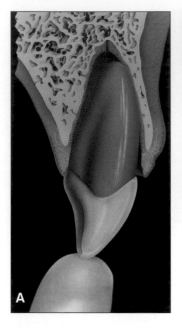
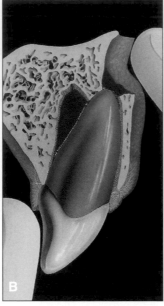
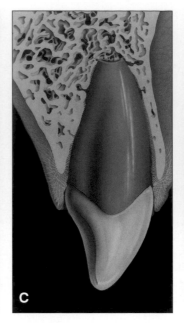
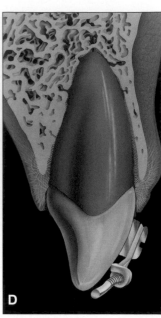

EFFECT OF REPOSITIONING

Depending on the force needed to reposition the tooth, more or less additional trauma will be transmitted to the periodontium and the pulp. Besides the need for repositioning with respect to occlusion and esthetics, this negative effect should be assessed in the light of possible benefits in subsequent wound healing of the approximation of wound surfaces. In the following, an outline is presented of the known effects of repositioning upon pulpal and periodontal wound healing.

PDL: incomplete – in contrast to complete – repositioning leads to a slight delay (approximately 2 weeks) in wound healing.[15,16] However, the end result for the PDL is the same. If part of the root surface is exposed to saliva (e.g. extrusive luxation), a loss of attachment in that particular region will occur unless complete repositioning is performed (A). In lateral luxation, the value of repositioning is not known (B). Especially in those cases where forceful repositioning is necessary, spontaneous

readjustment (in young individuals) or orthodontic readjustment should be considered. Occlusal and/or esthetic demands, however, usually require immediate repositioning even in these cases.

After intrusion of permanent teeth, spontaneous re-eruption can usually only be expected in teeth with incomplete root formation (C). In teeth with completed root formation, orthodontic re-eruption is possibly to be preferred over immediate repositioning (after the age of 12 years) in order to enhance marginal bone healing (D). However, there is no definite information yet available concerning this issue.

Pulp: optimal repositioning leads to a more rapid and more predictable pulpal revascularization.[15] Furthermore, if root formation is not complete, there is a good chance of survival of the epithelial root sheath and thereby an optimal chance of continued root growth.[15]

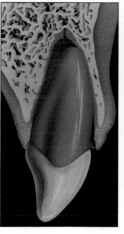
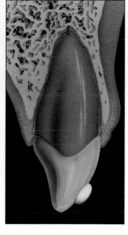

EFFECT OF SPLINTING

PDL: with a simple rupture of the PDL (e.g. extrusive luxation), rigid splinting does not promote healing.[16] Flexible splinting presently is assumed to assist periodontal healing, but this effect is not definitely proven. In situations with massive PDL cell death (e.g. avulsions), prolonged rigid splinting apparently leads to maintenance of initially formed ankylosis sites along the root surface. In these cases, short-term semi-rigid splinting (i.e. 1 week to permit initial endodontics) appears to be the treatment of choice. Semi-rigid and rigid splinting are discussed later (see page 56).

Pulp: rigid splinting appears to slow down pulpal revascularization. Nonsplinting or flexible splinting is to be preferred (see page 56).

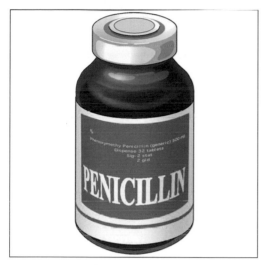

EFFECT OF ANTIBIOTICS

PDL: under experimental conditions, antibiotics administered either topically for 5 min before replantation of teeth in monkeys or systemically on the day of replantation have been found to decrease the extent of external root resorption.[23–26] The explanation for this is most likely the killing of bacteria on the root surface which must otherwise be eliminated by an inflammatory response, perhaps leading to an osteoclastic attack on the root surface (see page 12).

Pulp: the effect of antibiotics on pulpal healing is yet to be determined. Systemic administration of antibiotics after luxations or root fractures, has not been found in clinical studies to enhance pulpal healing; nor could any effect be seen experimentally after replantation of extracted teeth in monkeys.[27] However, experimental studies in monkeys has shown that a 5-min topical application of antibiotics (doxycycline, 1 mg in 20 ml physiologic saline) was found to favor the likelihood of revascularization after replantation of extracted teeth with immature root formation.[23,28] It should also be noted that a negative effect on healing following root fractures has been noted.[70]

NOTES

Classification of Dental Injuries

Dental injuries have been classified according to a variety of factors, such as etiology, anatomy, pathology, or therapeutic considerations.[29] The present classification is based on a system adopted by the World Health Organization (WHO) in its *Application of International Classification of Diseases to Dentistry and Stomatology*.[30] However, for the sake of completeness, it was felt necessary to define and classify certain trauma entities not included in the WHO system. The following classification includes injuries to the teeth, supporting structures, gingiva, and oral mucosa and is based on anatomical, therapeutic and prognostic considerations. This classification can be applied to both the permanent and the primary dentitions. The code number is according to the International Classification of Diseases (1995).[30]

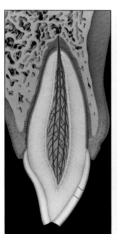
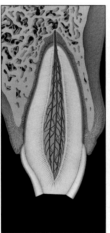
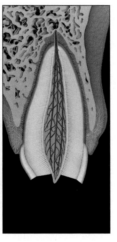

INJURIES TO THE HARD DENTAL TISSUES AND THE PULP

Enamel infraction (S 02.50). An incomplete fracture (crack) of the enamel without loss of tooth substance.

Enamel fracture (uncomplicated crown fracture) (S 02.50). A fracture with loss of tooth substance confined to the enamel.

Enamel–dentin fracture (uncomplicated crown fracture) (S 02.51). A fracture with loss of tooth substance confined to enamel and dentin, but not involving the pulp.

Complicated crown fracture (S 02.52). A fracture involving enamel and dentin, and exposing the pulp.

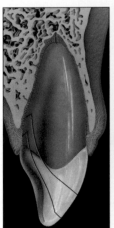
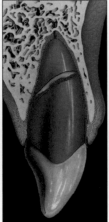
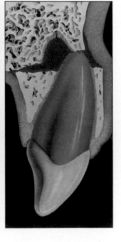

INJURIES TO THE HARD DENTAL TISSUES: THE PULP AND ALVEOLAR PROCESS

Crown-root fracture (S 02.54). A fracture involving enamel, dentin and cementum. It may or may not expose the pulp (uncomplicated and complicated crown-root fracture).

Root fracture (S 02.53). A fracture involving dentin, cementum, and the pulp. Root fractures can be further classified according to displacement of the coronal fragment (see luxation injuries).

Fracture of the mandibular (S 02.60) or **maxillary** (S 02.40) **alveolar socket wall**. A fracture of the alveolar process which involves the alveolar socket (see lateral luxation).

Fracture of the mandibular (S 02.60) or **maxillary** (S 02.40) **alveolar process**. A fracture of the alveolar process that may or may not involve the alveolar socket.

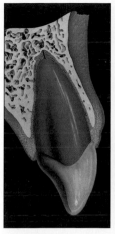
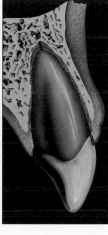
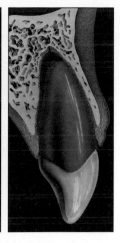

INJURIES TO THE PERIODONTAL TISSUES
(SEE ALSO PAGE 75)

Concussion (S 03.20). An injury to the tooth-supporting structures without abnormal loosening or displacement of the tooth, but with marked reaction to percussion.

Subluxation (loosening) (S 03.20). An injury to the tooth supporting structures with abnormal loosening, but without displacement of the tooth.

Extrusive luxation (peripheral dislocation, partial avulsion) (S 03.21). Partial displacement of the tooth out of its socket.

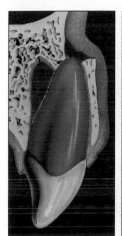
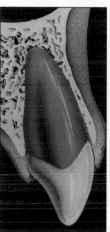
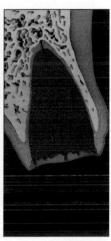

INJURIES TO THE PERIODONTAL TISSUES

Lateral luxation (S 03.20). Displacement of the tooth in a direction other than axially. This is accompanied by comminution or fracture of the alveolar socket.

Intrusive luxation (central dislocation) (S 03.21). Displacement of the tooth into the alveolar bone. This injury is accompanied by comminution or fracture of the alveolar socket.

Avulsion (exarticulation) (S 03.22). Complete displacement of the tooth out of its socket.

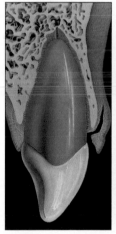
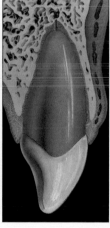
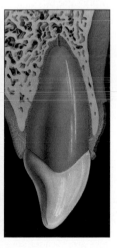

INJURIES TO GINGIVA OR ORAL MUCOSA

Laceration of gingiva or oral mucosa (S 01.50). A shallow or deep wound in the mucosa resulting from a tear; usually produced by a sharp object.

Contusion of gingiva or oral mucosa (S 01.50). A bruise usually produced by impact with a blunt object and not accompanied by a break in the mucosa, usually causing submucosal hemorrhage.

Abrasion of gingiva or oral mucosa (S 01.50). A superficial wound produced by rubbing or scraping of the mucosa, leaving a raw, bleeding surface.

NOTES

_____
_____
_____
_____
_____
_____

Examination and Diagnosis

OBJECTIVES

1 Perform clinical procedures to gather necessary information about the type and extent of injury.

2 Perform radiographic examination procedures to gather necessary information about injuries to the tooth and supporting structures.

3 Perform radiographic examination procedures to reveal foreign bodies embedded in lip wounds.

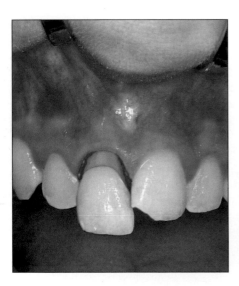 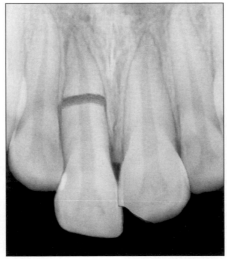 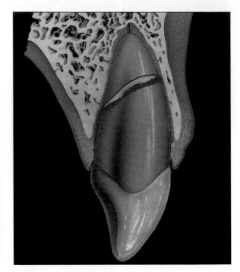

In order to arrive at a quick and correct diagnosis of the probable extent of injury to the pulp, periodontium and associated structures, a systematic examination of the traumatized patient is essential (see also Appendices 1–3).[31–33]

When the patient is received for treatment of an acute trauma, the oral region is usually heavily contaminated. The first step in the examination procedure, therefore, is to wash the patient's face. If there are soft tissue wounds, a mild detergent should be used. While this is being done, it is possible to get an initial impression of the extent of injury. Thereafter, a series of questions must be asked to aid in diagnosis and treatment planning. These questions include the following.

When did the injury occur?
The answer will imply a time factor, which is critical when considering avulsed or displaced teeth and could influence the choice of treatment.

Where did the injury occur?
While there might be legal implications in this answer, this will also indicate the possibility of contamination of wounds.

How did the injury occur?
The answer to this question will indicate possible zones of injury (e.g. crown-root fractures in the premolar and molar region after impact to the chin). Any inconsistency between the wounds observed on a child and the history supplied should raise the suspicion of child abuse and call for the assistance of other medical specialties. Also a marked treatment delay should raise the suspicion of child abuse.

Was there a period of unconsciousness?
If so, how long? Is there headache? Amnesia? Nausea? Vomiting? These are all signs of brain concussion and require medical attention. However, this usually does not contraindicate immediate treatment of the dental injury.

Have there been previous injuries to the teeth?
Answers to this may explain radiographic findings, such as pulp canal obliteration and incomplete root formation in a dentition with otherwise completed root development.

Is there disturbance in the bite?
An affirmative answer could imply tooth luxation, alveolar fracture, jaw fracture, or luxation or fracture of the temporomandibular joint.

Is there any reaction in the teeth to cold and/or heat?
A positive finding indicates exposure of dentin and need of dentinal coverage.

Medical history
Finally, a short medical history should reveal possible allergies, blood disorders and other information that may influence treatment.

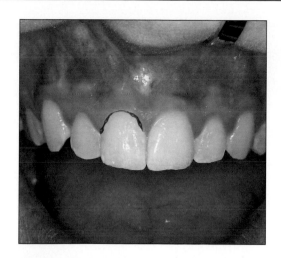

CLINICAL EXAMINATION

The first step in an adequate examination of the traumatized patient should be registration of clinical findings. Appendices 1 and 2 show standardized clinical examination forms that will aid the clinician in an orderly examination sequence and will ensure registration of all pertinent clinical information. The clinical examination should include examination of soft tissue wounds. If present, the penetrating nature of these should be determined, with emphasis on the possible presence of foreign bodies (see page 20). Thereafter, the hard dental tissues are examined for the presence of **infractions** and **fractures**. Directing the examination light beam parallel to the labial surface of the injured tooth facilitates the diagnosis of **infractions**. In cases of crown fractures, pulp exposures should be detected and their size noted. Moreover, concomitant luxation injuries should be recorded, as these have a negative influence on long-term prognosis with respect to pulpal healing.

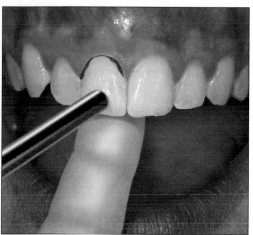

MOBILITY TEST

Mobility testing should determine the extent of loosening, especially axially, of individual teeth (an indication of disrupted pulpal vascularity) and mobility of groups of teeth (an indication of alveolar fracture). The **degree of mobility** is registered on a scale of 0–3 (0 = no loosening, 1 = horizontal loosening ≥ 1 mm, 2 = horizontal loosening ≥ 1 mm, 3 = axial loosening); and is an aid in defining the type of luxation.[32] It should be noted, however, that '0' mobility can either be physiological mobility or no mobility whatsoever, a sign of intrusion or lateral luxation at the time of injury, or ankylosis in the follow-up period. '0' mobility should, therefore, be used in conjunction with **percussion tone** for the definition of luxation injuries (see below).

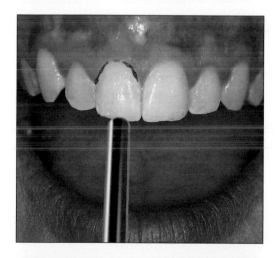

PERCUSSION TEST

Percussion testing, with a finger in small children or the handle of a metal instrument, has two functions. **Tenderness to percussion** will indicate damage to the PDL. Percussion of the labial surface will yield either a high or low **percussion tone**. A high, metallic tone implies that the injured tooth is locked into bone (as in lateral luxation or intrusion). At the follow-up examinations, this tone indicates ankylosis. This finding can be confirmed if a finger is placed on the oral surface of the tooth to be tested. It is possible to feel the tapping of the instrument on a tooth with a normal PDL. In cases of intrusion, lateral luxation or ankylosis, percussion cannot be felt through the tooth tested.

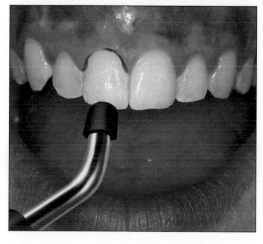

PULPAL SENSIBILITY TEST

Electrometric sensibility testing should be carried out whenever possible as it yields important information about the neurovascular supply to the pulp of involved teeth.[31,33] The most reliable response is obtained when the electrode is placed on the incisal edge or the most incisal aspect of enamel (with crown fractures). It should be noted that young teeth with incomplete root formation do not respond consistently to sensibility testing and at higher threshold values compared to teeth with completed root formation. However, the response at the time of injury provides a baseline value for comparison at later follow-up examinations. Finally, sensibility testing in the primary dentition may yield inconclusive information due to a lack of patient cooperation.

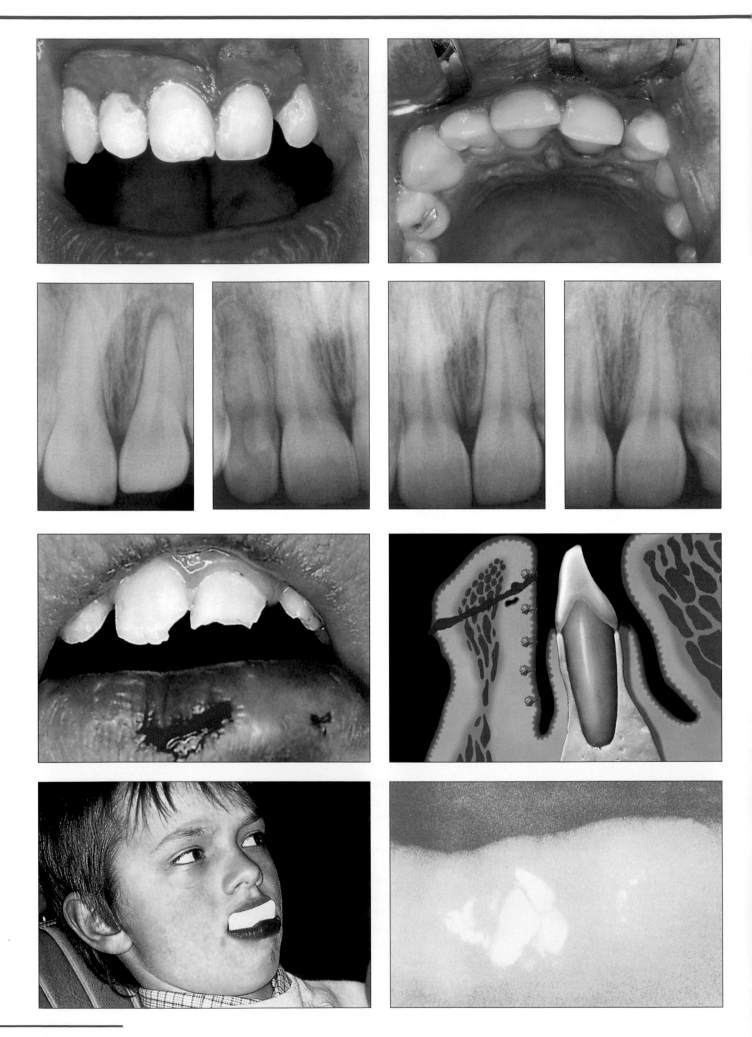

RADIOGRAPHIC EXAMINATION

The clinical examination, which has focused on the area of injury, is followed by a radiographic examination.

Several studies have demonstrated the importance of multiple radiographic exposures for revealing tooth displacement at the time of injury as well as periapical pathosis at the follow-up visits.[31-33] Radiographic film format is worth considering in order to achieve high quality, reproducible images. A steep occlusal exposure (using a size 2 film (DF 58, EP 21)) of the traumatized anterior region gives an excellent view of most **lateral luxations, apical and mid-root fractures and alveolar fractures**. The standard periapical bisecting angle exposure of each traumatized tooth (using a size 1 film (DF 56, EP 11)) provides information about **cervical root fractures** as well as other tooth displacements. Thus, a radiographic examination comprising one steep occlusal exposure and three periapical bisecting angle exposures of the traumatized region will provide sufficient information in determining the extent of trauma.

RADIOGRAPHIC EXAMINATION OF SOFT TISSUE LESIONS

In the presence of a **penetrating lip lesion**, a soft tissue radiograph is indicated in order to locate any foreign bodies.[31] It should be noted that the orbicularis oris muscles close tightly around foreign bodies in the lip, making them impossible to palpate; they can only be identified radiographically. This is accomplished by placing a dental film between the lips and the dental arch and using 25% of the normal exposure time. If this exposure reveals foreign bodies (a radiographic examination will normally demonstrate foreign bodies such as tooth fragments, composite filling material, metal, gravel, whereas organic materials such as cloth and wood cannot be seen), a lateral radiograph can be added (at 50% normal exposure time) to visualize the foreign bodies in relation to the cutaneous and mucosal surfaces of the lips. With the combined information from the clinical and radiographic examinations, diagnosis, prognosis and treatment planning can then be accomplished.

Finally, **photographic registration** of the trauma is recommended, as it offers an exact documentation of the extent of injury and can be used later in treatment planning, legal claims or clinical research.

FOLLOW-UP

A well-designed follow up procedure is essential to diagnose complications. The following recall schedule has been found suitable in this regard:

- **1 week** (only for patients with replanted teeth). A splint should usually be removed at this time to prevent ankylosis.

- **3 weeks**. A radiographic examination is able to demonstrate periapical radiolucency as well as in some instances inflammatory resorption. After luxation, the splint can usually be removed.

- **6 weeks**. A clinical and radiographic examination is able to demonstrate most cases of pulp necrosis as well as inflammatory root resorption.

- **2 and 6 months**. Optional for cases with questionable healing.

- **1 year**. A clinical and radiographic examination can ascertain the long-term prognosis. Special trauma entities such as root fractures, intrusions, and replanted teeth may require longer observation periods.

NOTES

Diagnosis of Pulpal Healing Complications

OBJECTIVES

1 Recognize the clinical and radiographic signs of pulp healing, pulp necrosis, and pulp canal obliteration.

2 Identify time periods after trauma where these healing events can be diagnosed.

3 Recognize the existence of transient apical breakdown.

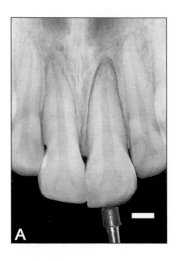 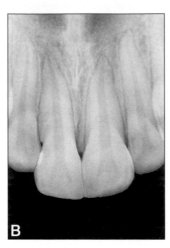 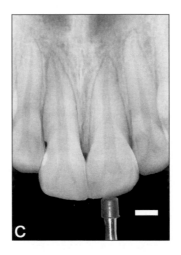 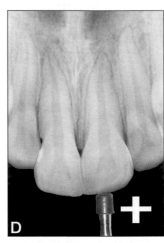

PULP HEALING

After a luxation injury, there may be partial or total disruption of the neurovascular supply apically. In case of partial disruption, reduced circulation can still be maintained throughout the pulp, with complete reconstitution of the neurovasculature after a few weeks. In cases of total rupture of the neurovascular supply, gradual revascularization will take place in an apico-coronal direction at a rate of approximately 0.5 mm vessel ingrowth per day.[34] Signs of successful revascularization are a narrowing of the pulp canal and positive sensibility testing which usually takes place after 2–3 months (A–D).

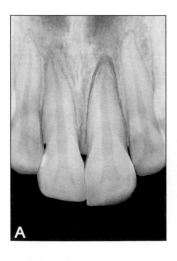 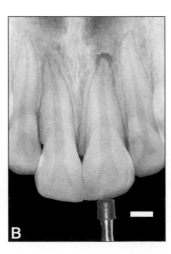 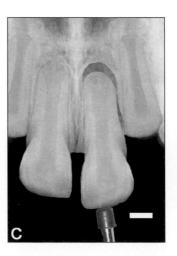 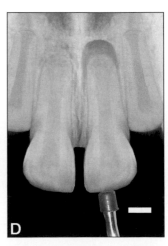

PULP NECROSIS

In cases where the injury has implied a partial or total rupture of the neurovascular supply, revascularization and reinnervation processes will be initiated. Whether these processes succeed depends primarily on two factors: (1) the size of the apical foramen and (2) the presence of bacteria in the healing site.[34–36] Unsuccessful pulp healing with an infected pulp is evident radiographically as periapical radiolucency, usually after 2–4 weeks (B and D). In rare cases, a sterile necrosis may occur; and in these cases there will be no radiolucency. The classical signs of pulp necrosis (PN) are discoloration of the crown (gray, blue or red), negative sensibility testing, apical radiolucency, as well as persistent tenderness to percussion. Moreover, with immature teeth, PN can be seen as arrested root development, with or without apical closure. If two or more signs of PN are present, pulp extirpation is usually indicated.

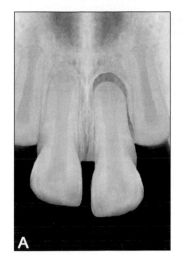

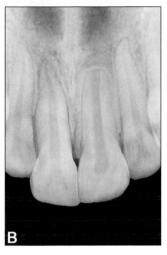

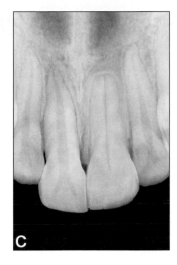

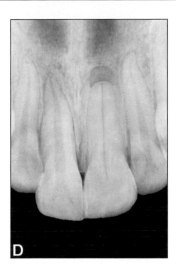

PULP CANAL OBLITERATION

In cases where the injury causes severance of the neurovascular supply of the pulp, healing implies revascularization and reinnervation of the ischemic pulp (see page 11). If this process succeeds, hard tissue deposition along the pulp canal walls resumes; however at an accelerated pace.[37–39] This type of pulp response is frequent in all types of luxation injuries with displacement. Within 1 year, an almost totally obliterated pulp canal may be seen (A–C). Such a tooth runs a 1% annual risk of developing pulp necrosis (D).[37–39] The cause for this has not yet been determined.

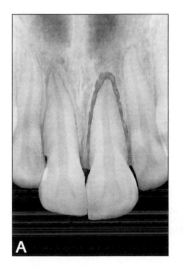

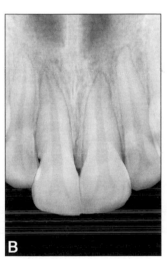

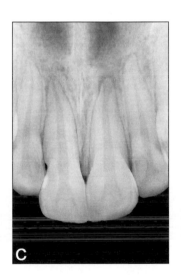

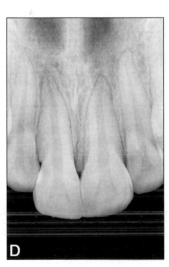

TRANSIENT APICAL BREAKDOWN

Where the injury has implied severance of the neurovascular supply and the apical foramen is narrow, the revascularization process will also engage osteoclastic activity in the base of the socket and the root canal opening in order to make room for ingrowth of new tissue (A–C).[40] This process is transient; and when revascularization is complete, the radiolucent area will disappear (D). This process is usually seen 2–12 months after injury and usually involves extruded and laterally luxated young permanent teeth.

NOTES

_____

_____

_____

_____

_____

_____

Diagnosis of Periodontal Healing Complications

OBJECTIVES

1 Recognize the radiographic signs of the three resorption types which may affect the root surface after trauma.

2 Identify time periods after trauma when the different resorption types are likely to occur.

3 Recognize the existence of transient marginal breakdown.

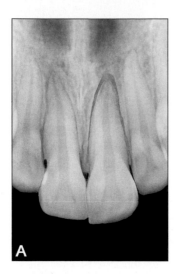 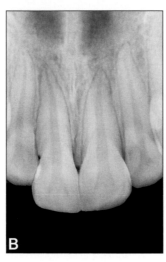 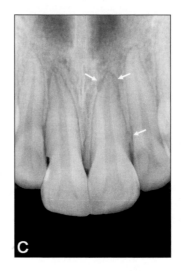 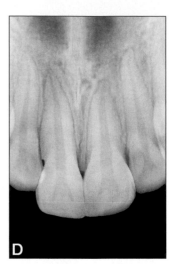

REPAIR-RELATED RESORPTION (SURFACE RESORPTION)

This resorption entity represents the healing response to a localized injury in the PDL, affecting the cells next to the root surface (see page 12). The typical situation where repair-related resorption occurs appears to be concussion and lateral luxation (A–D).[41–43] It can also occur following intrusion and replantation, where it may affect all parts of the root, and in root fractures, where it is seen next to the fracture line.[42–46] Repair-related resorption is typically diagnosed 4 weeks after injury.

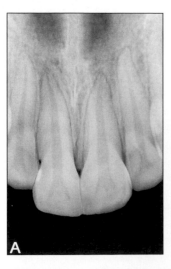 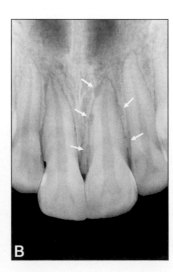 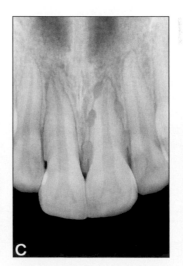 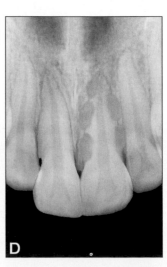

INFECTION-RELATED RESORPTION (INFLAMMATORY RESORPTION)

This resorption entity represents a combined injury to the pulp and PDL, and where bacteria primarily located in the pulp canal and dentinal tubules trigger osteoclastic activity on the root surface (see page 12). This type of resorption can affect all parts of the root and is especially common after intrusion and replantation of avulsed teeth. Infection-related resorption is typically diagnosed 2–4 weeks after injury.[42,43,115] This resorption is a rapidly progressing process which may result in total resorption of the root after a month (A–D).

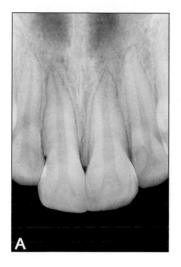 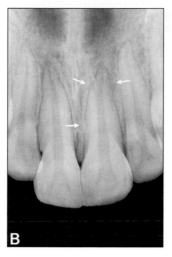 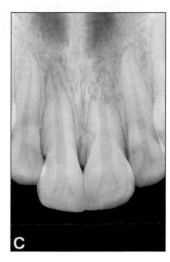 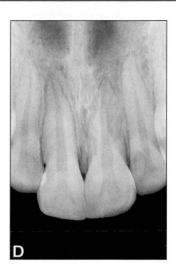

ANKYLOSIS-RELATED RESORPTION (REPLACEMENT RESORPTION)

This resorption process is in response to extensive damage to the innermost layer of the PDL. Due to the predominant healing response from the socket wall, an ankylosis is formed (see page 13). Because of the remodeling characteristic of bone, the root structure is gradually replaced by bone (A–D).[46,115] Ankylosis is frequent after intrusion and replantation of avulsed teeth. It can usually be diagnosed radiographically 2 months after injury; but clinically after 1 month (i.e. high percussion sound).

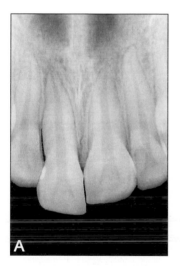 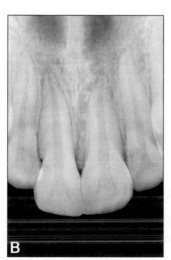 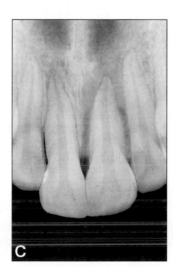 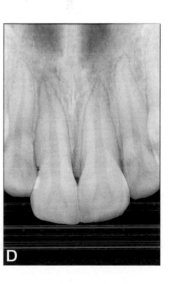

TRANSIENT MARGINAL BREAKDOWN

Where there has been extensive damage to the bony part of the socket, resorption of the injured socket wall must take place prior to healing. This event may occur after lateral luxation and intrusion; and can be seen radiographically as resorption of the lamina dura and clinically as granulation tissue in the gingival area. After 1 month, this process will resolve with later reformation of socket bone (A–D).

NOTES

_____

_____

_____

_____

_____

_____

Treatment Priorities of Dental Trauma

OBJECTIVE 1 To define trauma conditions, which should be treated acutely (i.e. within a few hours), subacutely (i.e. within 24 hours) or delayed (i.e. after 24 hours).

ACUTE APPROACH

It has commonly been accepted that all injuries should be treated on an emergency basis. This is for the comfort of the patient and also to reduce wound healing complications. For practical, and especially economic reasons, various approaches can be selected to fulfill such a demand, such as acute (i.e. within a few hours), subacute (i.e. within the first 24 hours), and delayed treatment (i.e. after the first 24 hours). The following classification into these three categories is based on a recent study of the effect of treatment delay on the various trauma entities.[47]

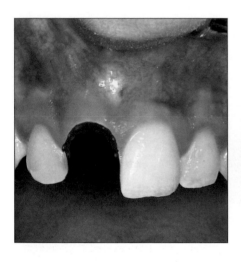 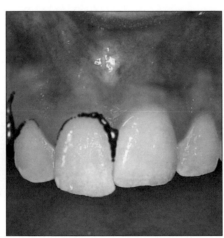

TOOTH AVULSION

A very strong relationship has been found between healing outcome and storage condition and storage time (see page 50). This should therefore be considered an acute trauma situation, at least if the tooth has not been replanted.

ALVEOLAR FRACTURE

In one clinical study a significant relationship was found between the occurrence of pulp necrosis and treatment delay for more than 3 hours.[47]

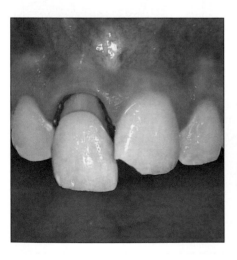 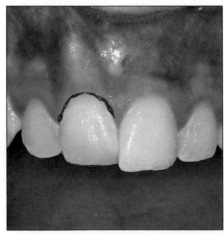 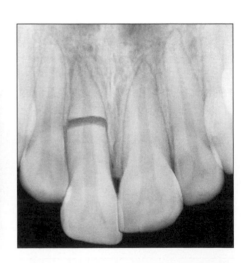

EXTRUSION, LATERAL LUXATION AND ROOT FRACTURE

At present there are only a few studies that have examined the effect of treatment delay on pulpal healing after luxation injuries and root fractures. One study of luxated teeth has shown a significant difference in healing after a treatment delay of 5 hours. Other studies have shown a difference between treatment delays for 33 hours and more.[47] A recent study of 455 root fractures could not verify an effect of early treatment. Until new research shows otherwise, these traumas should be considered candidates for acute treatment.

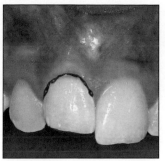

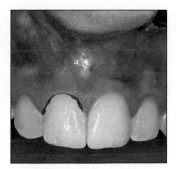

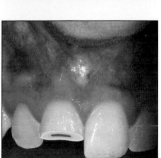

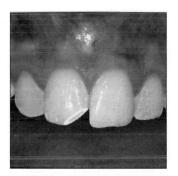

SUBACUTE APPROACH

Intrusion

A recent clinical study has shown almost identical healing results of immediate (surgical) repositioning and delayed orthodontic repositioning. It therefore seems reasonable to use a subacute approach for this trauma entity.[49]

Concussion, subluxation

A clinical study could not demonstrate a relationship between immediate treatment and pulp complications. A subacute treatment approach is therefore acceptable.[47]

Crown fractures with pulp exposure

Recent clinical studies have shown that crown fractures with pulp exposure have the same long-term prognosis whether treated on an acute, subacute or delayed basis. Due to the discomfort of an exposed pulp, a subacute treatment approach is therefore indicated.[47]

Primary teeth

Primary teeth can probably be treated with a subacute or delayed strategy unless occlusal interference due to tooth displacement indicates an acute approach to relieve symptoms.

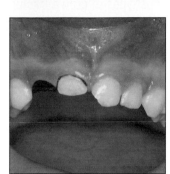

DELAYED TREATMENT

Crown fractures without pulp exposure

Recent studies of crown fractures without pulp exposure have shown the same prognosis whether treated on an acute, subacute or delayed basis. A subacute or delayed approach is therefore acceptable.[47]

NOTES

_____

_____

_____

_____

_____

_____

Crown Fracture without Pulp Exposure

OBJECTIVES

1 Based on clinical findings, differentiate between the types of fractures: infractions, enamel, enamel–dentin without pulpal involvement.
2 Make treatment decisions based on such factors as the extent of injury, development of the tooth, status of the pulp.
3 Provide appropriate treatment for the various types of crown fractures.
4 Recognize crown fracture situations that permit fragment reattachment.

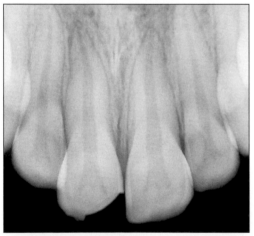

DEFINITIONS AND CLINICAL APPEARANCE

Infraction is a disruption of enamel prisms without loss of tooth substance that extends from the enamel surface to the dentino–enamel junction. **Enamel fracture** is the loss of tooth substance confined to enamel. **Enamel–dentin fracture** (uncomplicated crown fracture) is the loss of tooth substance confined to enamel and dentin, but not involving the pulp.

Fractures may appear as a crazing within the enamel or as loss of tooth substance involving only enamel or enamel and dentin. Infraction lines are usually best seen when the light beam is directed parallel to the long axis of the tooth. Besides describing only the most obvious injury (i.e. crown fracture), it is very important to diagnose concomitant luxation injuries, as these have significant influence on pulpal outcome (see pages 38–47).

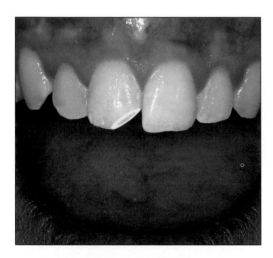

RADIOGRAPHIC APPEARANCE

The lost part of the crown can usually be recognized, whereas infraction lines cannot be seen.

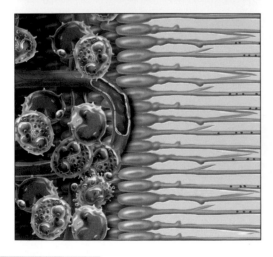

BIOLOGIC CONSIDERATIONS AND TREATMENT PRINCIPLES

Exposed dentinal tubules can permit invasion of bacteria or bacterial toxins to the pulp and result in pulpal inflammation.[50] The severity of this response is related to pulpal vascularity, i.e. whether or not the neurovascular supply has been compromised by a concomitant luxation injury (see page 11).

Treatment principally consists of protecting the pulp from external insults and restoring normal function and esthetics. If there is no associated periodontal injury (luxation), the tooth can be restored immediately using resin composites and dental adhesives. In cases of concomitant luxation injury associated with tooth mobility and gingival bleeding, a temporary restoration is indicated, as a dry operative field is difficult to maintain. In these cases, care must be taken that the temporary material is not forced into the ruptured periodontal ligament space.

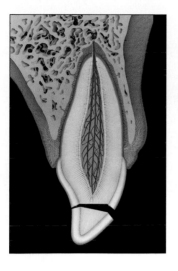 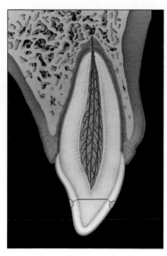 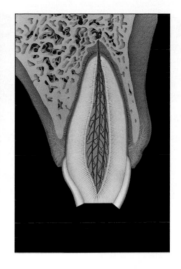 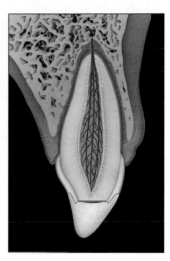

TREATMENT AND POSTOPERATIVE CONTROL

In cases of superficial enamel fractures, selective grinding of the injured tooth may be the only treatment necessary.

If a crown fragment is retrieved and without significant substance loss, it can be reattached using dental adhesives and resin composites.[50,51] Whether resin composite build-up or fragment reattachment is the treatment of choice, a dental adhesive should be employed. A recent laboratory study has demonstrated that bonding strength equal to that of intact teeth can be achieved with the new bonding systems.[52]

After fragment reattachment, optimal esthetics are achieved if the fracture line labially is prepared with a double chamfer and restored with resin composite.

When using resin composite build-up, optimal esthetics and function are achieved when the fracture edges are prepared with a 1–2 mm wide chamfer margin prior to build-up.

In cases where neither of these treatments can be performed, an emergency procedure comprises application of a provisional bandage consisting of glass ionomer cement.

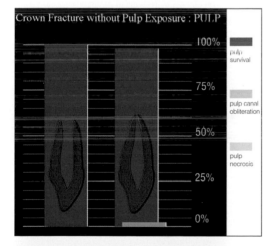

EXPECTED OUTCOME: PULP

The tooth should be monitored 2 months after injury. If sensibility is normal, no further control is indicated. In cases of concomitant luxation injuries, controls follow those recommended for the respective injury category.

The risk of pulpal complications is minimal.[51,53–58] However, the risk of pulp necrosis is significantly enhanced in the case of additional luxation injury. Thus, it appears that the luxation diagnosis alone determines the risk of pulp necrosis.

The graphs show pulp outcome for crown fractures without luxation injuries.

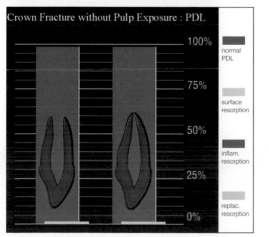

EXPECTED OUTCOME: PDL

Periodontal complications are extremely rare after crown fractures and consist only of surface resorption.[56,58]

Crown Fracture with Pulp Exposure

OBJECTIVES
1. Recognize tissue changes resulting from pulp exposure and concomitant luxation injuries.
2. Determine treatment options.
3. Provide emergency and definitive care.

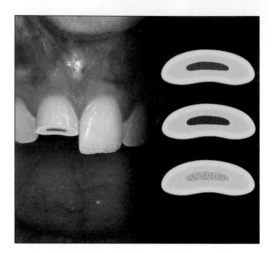

DEFINITION AND CLINICAL APPEARANCE

A fracture involving enamel and dentin, and exposing the pulp (complicated crown fracture).

Depending on the absence or presence of a concomitant luxation injury, the pulp will present with a bright red, cyanotic or ischemic appearance, respectively. There may be spontaneous bleeding from the pulp.

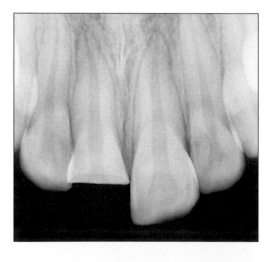

RADIOGRAPHIC APPEARANCE

Lost tooth substance is apparent, as well as periodontal changes in the case of concomitant luxation.

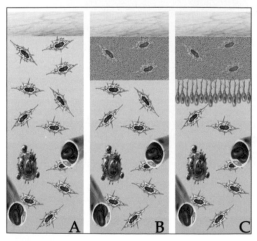

BIOLOGIC CONSIDERATIONS

Exposed dentinal tubules and the exposed pulp allow indirect and direct insult to the pulp, which responds with an inflammatory response and subsequent formation of granulation tissue.[59] Bacteria can penetrate exposed dentinal tubules and will also be found on the surface of the pulp. However, bacterial colonization is hindered if pulpal vascularity is intact.

When pulp capping or partial pulpotomy are performed (A) with calcium hydroxide as the amputation material (shaded area), the following healing events will occur.[59] Coagulation necrosis is seen in the tissue immediately beneath the calcium hydroxide (B). Immediately below this zone, a wound healing response will be seen whereby new odontoblasts are differentiated and begin to form new dentin (C). This occurs 2–3 weeks after treatment. At this time, up to 5 μm of new dentin can be deposited daily, which means that after 2–3 months, a significant hard tissue barrier has been formed under the pulpal wound.

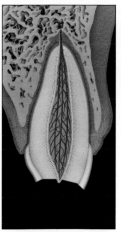
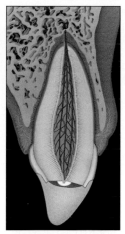

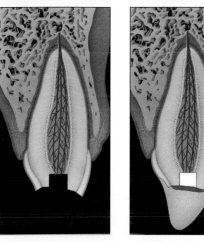

TREATMENT

A hard tissue barrier can be expected to be formed under the following conditions: normal pulp status prior to trauma; intact vascular supply to the pulp after trauma; the use of an appropriate pulp capping or amputation technique; and exclusion of bacteria in the pulp capping or pulp amputation zone during the healing period.[59] If the prognosis for pulp capping is not favorable, or the absence of the pulp is preferable (i.e. due to later crown restoration and/or the placement of a post), the pulp should be extirpated.

PULP CAPPING

The tooth is isolated with rubber dam and the fracture surface is cleaned with chlorhexidine and sodium hypochlorite. Calcium hydroxide paste is applied only to the pulpal wound. Thereafter, the tooth can be restored either with dentin adhesive and conventional resin composite build-up or fragment reattachment in the latter case space should be made in the coronal fragment for the amputation paste.[59] Radiographic evidence of hard tissue healing can be seen 3 months after treatment.

PARTIAL PULPOTOMY

The tooth is anesthetized, isolated with rubber dam and the fracture surface cleaned with chlorhexidine. Preferably using a round carbide bur or diamond mounted in an air rotor with copious water spray, the pulp is removed to a depth of 2–3 mm, creating a box-like cavity. Once complete hemostasis is achieved, a thin layer of calcium hydroxide paste or mineral trioxide aggregate (MTA) (see page 59) is applied to the wound and compressed slightly. Over this, and still within the prepared cavity, a thin layer of resin-modified glass ionomer cement is applied. Thereafter, the tooth can be restored using dental adhesive with either conventional resin composite build-up or crown fragment reattachment.[59] Radiographic examination should be made to detect signs of pulp necrosis or pulp canal obliteration (both rare findings in cases of fracture without concomitant luxation injury).

EXPECTED OUTCOME: PULP CAPPING

Long-term studies have shown very high success rates of pulp capping and partial pulpotomy with respect to pulp survival.[59-62]

Radiographic evidence of hard tissue closure of the perforation can be seen 3 months after treatment. The tooth should be followed 1 and 5 years after injury and monitored for pulpal sensibility. When using resin composite build-up, the pulp tester should be placed on the most incisal aspect of the available enamel.

The graphs show pulp outcome for crown fractures without luxation injuries.[60]

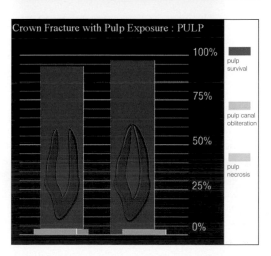

EXPECTED OUTCOME: PARTIAL PULPOTOMY

Long-term studies have shown very high success rates of partial pulpotomy with respect to pulp survival irrespective of the stage of root development.[62]

Crown-root Fracture

OBJECTIVES

1   Identify the tissues involved.
2   Provide emergency care to reduce pain due to mobile crown-root fragments.
3   Select appropriate treatment.

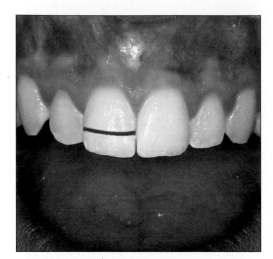

DEFINITION AND CLINICAL APPEARANCE

This is a fracture involving enamel, dentin and cementum, with or without pulpal involvement.

The fracture usually starts at the midportion of the crown facially and extends below the gingival level palatally. The coronal fragment is more or less displaced in an incisal direction, which results in pain from occlusion. In the premolar and molar regions, the fracture is usually confined to the buccal or oral cusps.

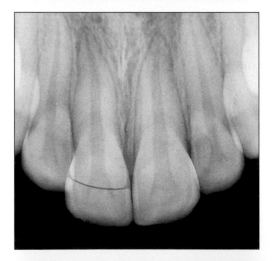

RADIOGRAPHIC APPEARANCE

With labio-lingual fractures only the incisal part of the fracture can be identified, whereas the lingual and more apically placed part of the fracture usually cannot be seen due to the hinge-like displacement of the fragment. Typically, proximal crown-root fractures are evident radiographically.

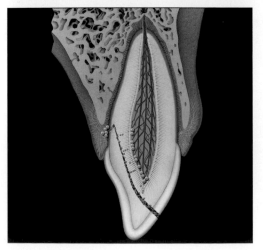

BIOLOGIC CONSIDERATIONS

The histologic events in the pulp mimic those of complicated and uncomplicated crown fractures, depending on the location of the fracture. Due to plaque accumulation in the line of fracture, the PDL next to the fracture line also shows inflammatory changes.[63]

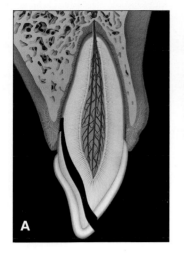 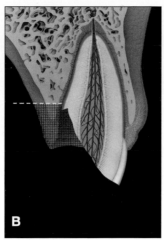 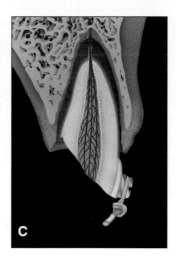 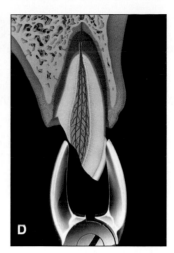

TREATMENT PRINCIPLES

The treatment principle is to seal exposed dentinal tubules and protect the pulp; to restore the tooth to original function and esthetics.[63]

The extent of the fracture below the gingival margin, as related to the length and morphology of the root, dictates the treatment chosen. The primary goal is to create a situation where the tooth can be restored after removal of the coronal fragment. In some cases, the apical fragment can be left in position and the tooth restored with or without exposing the subgingival aspect of the fracture; or the tooth can be surgically or orthodontically extruded into a position where restoration is possible. All forms of treatment can be performed either immediately or after some days' or weeks' delay. If treatment must be postponed, the coronal fragment can be temporarily splinted to adjacent teeth using an acid etch technique and composite resin. Immobilization of the loose fragment will be enough to alleviate symptoms and permit the patient to leave the emergency service free of pain.

FRAGMENT REMOVAL AND GINGIVAL REATTACHMENT (A)

The coronal fragment is removed and the gingiva is allowed to reattach to the exposed dentin (i.e. by formation of a long junctional epithelium). After some weeks, the tooth can be restored above the gingival level.

FRAGMENT REMOVAL AND SURGICAL EXPOSURE OF SUBGINGIVAL FRACTURE (B)

If the fracture extends below the alveolar crest, the subgingival fracture is exposed by gingivectomy and/or osteotomy after removal of the coronal fragment. Following gingival healing, the tooth is restored with a post-retained crown. While this procedure might appear to be most direct, long-term esthetic success can be compromised due to an accumulation of granulation tissue in the gingival sulcus palatally, which can lead to labial migration of the restored tooth.

FRAGMENT REMOVAL AND ORTHODONTIC EXTRUSION (C)

The coronal fragment is initially stabilized to adjacent teeth. Pulp extirpation and canal obturation with gutta percha and sealer can be performed at a later appointment. The coronal fragment is then removed and the tooth extruded over a 4–6-week period. The tooth should be slightly overextruded (0.5 mm), due to risk of relapse. A labial gingivectomy is performed, whereafter the tooth can be restored.

FRAGMENT REMOVAL AND SURGICAL EXTRUSION (D)

The coronal fragment is removed, whereafter the root is loosened with elevators and forceps and repositioned in a more incisal position, so that the entire fracture surface is exposed above the gingival level.[63–68] The root fragment is then stabilized with sutures or a nonrigid splint. The pulp is extirpated and the entrance to the root canal is sealed with temporary cement. After 4 weeks, when the tooth is stabilized in its socket, endodontic treatment is completed; and after another 4–5 weeks, the tooth can be restored.

TOOTH REMOVAL

Indicated in cases of fractures, which extend so deep below the gingival margin that the crown–root ratio after extrusion does not allow a crown restoration.

NOTES

_____

_____

_____

_____

_____

_____

Root Fracture

OBJECTIVES
1 Recognize the tissues involved.
2 Define objectives for acute treatment.
3 Describe healing outcomes based on a clinical and radiographic evaluation.
4 Describe treatment options for healing complications.

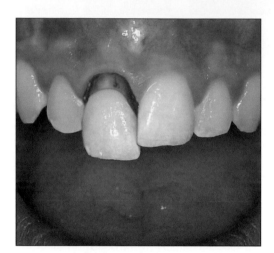

DEFINITION AND CLINICAL APPEARANCE

Root fractures are fractures involving dentin, cementum and the pulp. Root fractures can be further classified according to displacement of the coronal fragment (see under luxation injuries on page 17). Clinically, the tooth appears elongated and is usually displaced palatally.

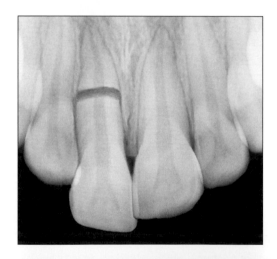

RADIOGRAPHIC APPEARANCE

Radiolucent line(s) separate the root into two or more fragments. The apical fragment is always left *in situ*, whereas the coronal fragment is often displaced. It should be noted that in cases where there is minimal luxation (i.e. concussion, subluxation) of the coronal fragment, the root fracture may not be evident until a later radiographic examination.

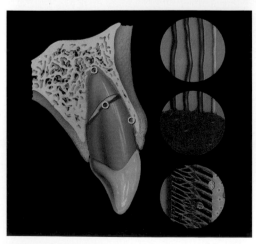

BIOLOGIC CONSIDERATIONS AND TREATMENT PRINCIPLES

This is a complex injury to the PDL, pulp, dentin and cementum. The injury to the coronal segment can be considered a luxation injury, with resultant trauma to the PDL and neurovascular supply to the coronal pulp. In contrast, the apical fragment remains essentially uninjured.[69] To facilitate healing, optimal repositioning is considered essential. The effect of firm splinting as well as the length of splinting time is presently not known, but under investigation.

In cases of root fracture with associated luxation, the displaced coronal fragment should be gently repositioned. This procedure is usually not painful, rarely indicating the use of local anesthesia. After repositioning, a control radiograph is taken. The tooth is then splinted. A rigid or semi-rigid splint can be used (see page 56).

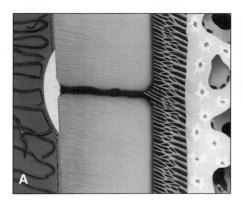
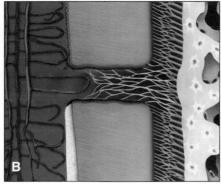
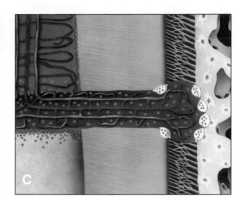

HEALING EVENTS AFTER ROOT FRACTURE

Healing outcome after root fracture can be divided into three groups:

- **Hard tissue healing (HT)**, where dentin (from odontoblasts) and cementum (from the periodontium) bridge the fracture gap (A).

- **Connective tissue healing (CT)**, where PDL cells invade the entire fracture gap and enclose both fragments (B).

- **Interposition of granulation tissue (GT)**, when the coronal pulp becomes infected and necrotic via the initial break in the PDL. Granulation tissue is then formed between the two fragments as a response to the infected coronal root canal (C).[69,70] When GT is successfully treated endodontically (coronal fragment), optimally with a calcium hydroxide interim dressing followed by gutta percha root filling, healing will resolve as CT.[69,70]

The following clinical and radiographic signs can be recorded, which indicate type of healing:

- **HT:** normal tooth mobility, normal pulpal sensibility, slightly discernible fracture line and an intact coronal pulp canal radiographically.

- **CT:** increased mobility of the involved tooth, normal pulpal sensibility, markedly discernible fracture line and obliteration of the coronal pulp canal radiographically.

- **GT:** increased to excessive mobility of the involved tooth, sometimes extrusion, negative pulpal sensibility, increasing radiographic distance between fragments and bone resorption (radiolucency) at the level of fracture.[71,72]

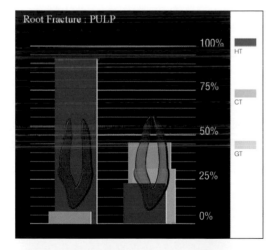

EXPECTED OUTCOME: PULP

The most significant factor determining healing events appears to be the stage of root development at the time of injury and the extent of initial displacement (luxation) of the coronal fragment.[70–81] In immature teeth, healing with HT is very frequent, whereas in mature teeth, healing by CT and nonhealing with GT predominate.[72,79] Moreover, HT is related to fractures with an intact pulp from the time of injury (concussion, subluxation). CT is related to moderate pulpal damage due to minor displacement of the coronal fragment (extrusion, lateral luxation) and in cases of incomplete repositioning.[70]

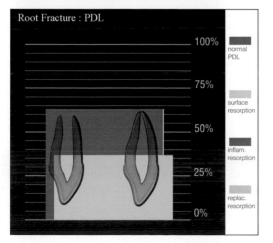

EXPECTED OUTCOME: PDL

Resorptions within the coronal pulp canal next to the fracture line can often be seen as steps in the HT and CT healing process and should not be confused with GT.[71,72]

Fracture of the Alveolar Process

OBJECTIVES
1. Recognize injury by appropriate clinical and radiographic techniques.
2. Identify the various dental and periodontal elements involved in the injury.
3. Define objectives of acute treatment.
4. Describe healing outcomes.

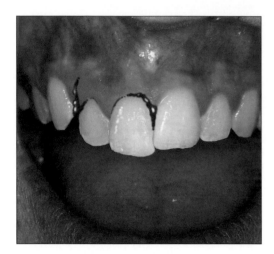

DEFINITION AND CLINICAL APPEARANCE

This trauma entity is defined as a fracture of the alveolar process, which may or may not involve the alveolar socket.

The typical clinical appearance is where a segment containing one or more teeth is displaced axially or laterally, usually resulting in occlusal disturbance. When mobility testing is performed, the entire fragment is found to be mobile, and percussion test gives a dull sound. Gingival lacerations are frequent.

RADIOGRAPHIC APPEARANCE

A fracture line can usually be seen, but depends on the angle of the central radiographic beam. The horizontal part of the fracture line may be found in all locations, ranging from the cervical to the apical or periapical region. A differential diagnosis must be made with root fracture. Change in the angulation of the central beam in a root fracture will not alter the fracture position on the root surface. However, the fracture line will move up or down in relation to the root surface according to angulation with cases of alveolar fracture.

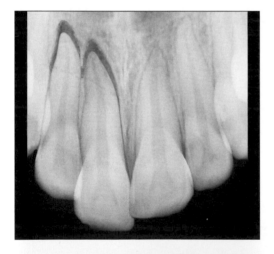

BIOLOGIC CONSIDERATIONS AND TREATMENT PRINCIPLES

The bony fracture may disrupt vascular supply to the associated teeth, which can result in pulp necrosis. Due to the frequent concomitant luxation injury and damage to the PDL, root resorption can sometimes occur.[82]

The treatment principles comprise repositioning and immobilization of the displaced bone–tooth fragment and monitoring of pulp vitality.

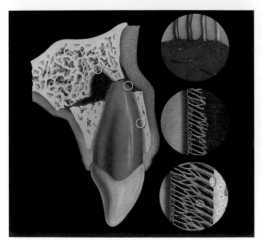

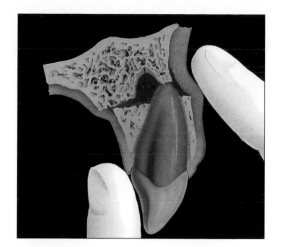

TREATMENT

Using infiltration or preferably a regional block anesthesia, the fragment is repositioned. As with lateral luxation, it is sometimes necessary to disengage the apices of the involved teeth from a bony lock. The fractured segment is splinted with a rigid or semi-rigid splint (see page 56).

The splint is removed after 3–4 weeks. Pulpal and PDL healing should be monitored after 4, 8 and 26 weeks and after 1 year.[83-84]

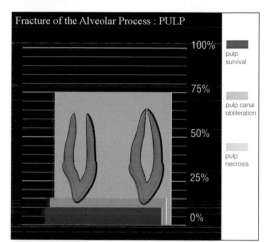

EXPECTED OUTCOME: PULP

Pulp necrosis is a frequent finding in root closed teeth.[83]

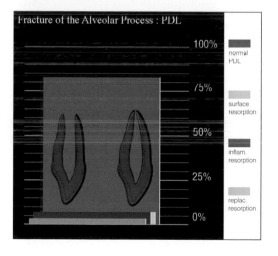

EXPECTED OUTCOME: PDL

Root resorption is a rare finding.[83]

NOTES

Concussion

OBJECTIVES
1. Differentiate type of luxation injury.
2. Identify injured tissues involved.
3. Define objectives of acute treatment.
4. Estimate frequency and type of possible complications.

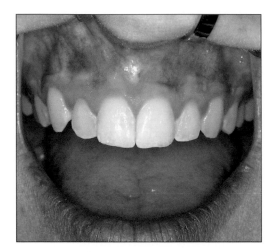

DEFINITION AND CLINICAL APPEARANCE

This lesion is defined as an injury to the tooth-supporting structures without abnormal loosening or displacement of the tooth. The only deviation from normal is a marked tenderness to percussion.

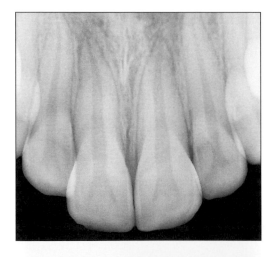

RADIOGRAPHIC APPEARANCE

The tooth is found in its normal position in the socket.

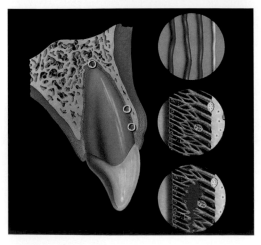

BIOLOGIC CONSIDERATIONS

The impact results in injury to the PDL, including edema and bleeding. Further effect of the impact may be damage to the neurovascular supply to the pulp.[85]

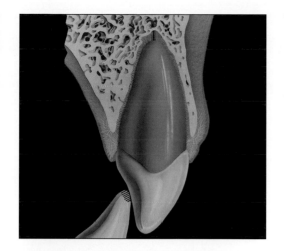

TREATMENT

If the tooth is in occlusion, the antagonist(s) can be slightly ground out of occlusion. The patient is placed on a soft diet for 2 weeks. Alternatively, the teeth can be splinted for patient comfort (approximately 2 weeks) or, with multiple tooth injuries, splinted according to the recommended fixation period for other injured teeth in the dental arch.

Only a few controls are indicated, for instance after 6 weeks and 1 year.

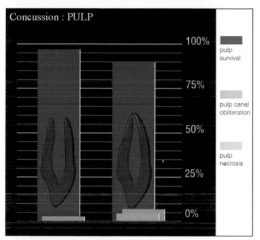

EXPECTED OUTCOME: PULP

Pulpal complications are rare. Stage of root development is the decisive prognostic factor.[86,87]

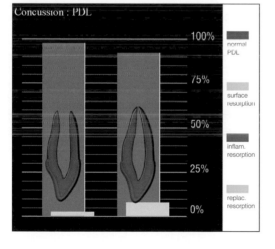

EXPECTED OUTCOME: PDL

Root resorption is very rare and consists exclusively in surface resorption.[86,89]

NOTES

Subluxation

OBJECTIVES
1 Differentiate type of luxation injury.
2 Identify injured tissues involved.
3 Define objectives of acute treatment.
4 Estimate frequency and type of complications.

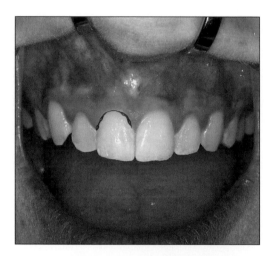

DEFINITIONS AND CLINICAL APPEARANCE

This luxation entity is an injury to the tooth-supporting structures with abnormal loosening, but without tooth displacement.

A subluxated tooth (right central incisor) is mobile and there might be hemorrhage from the gingival sulcus.

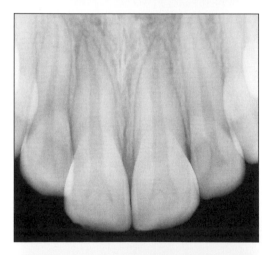

RADIOGRAPHIC APPEARANCE

The tooth is in its normal position in the socket.

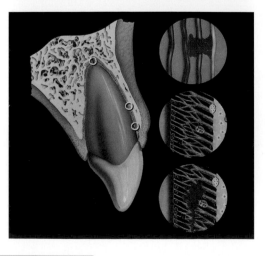

BIOLOGIC CONSIDERATIONS

The impact results in injury to the PDL, whereby edema, bleeding and tearing of PDL fibers may occur. A secondary effect of the impact may be total or partial rupture of the neurovascular supply to the pulp.[88]

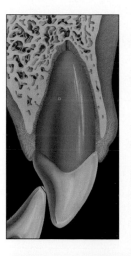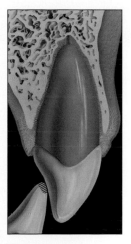

TREATMENT

If the tooth is in occlusion, the antagonist(s) can be slightly ground out of occlusion, and the patient is placed on a soft diet for 2 weeks. Alternatively, the teeth can be splinted for patient comfort (approximately 2 weeks) or, with of multiple tooth injuries, splinted according to the recommended fixation period for other injured tooth in the dental arch.

Only a few controls are indicated, for instance after 6 weeks and 1 year.

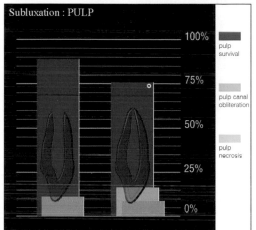

EXPECTED OUTCOME: PULP

Pulpal complications are rare. Stage of root development is the decisive prognostic factor.[89,90]

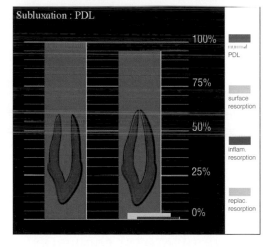

EXPECTED OUTCOME: PDL

Root resorption is very rare; and then primarily surface resorption.[90]

NOTES

Extrusive Luxation

OBJECTIVES

1 Differentiate type of luxation injury.
2 Identify injured tissues involved.
3 Define objectives of acute treatment.
4 Estimate frequency and type of complications.

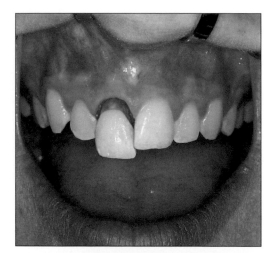

DEFINITION AND CLINICAL APPEARANCE
This lesion is defined as an injury whereby the tooth suffers axial displacement partially out of the socket.

The tooth appears elongated and is usually displaced palatally. The tooth is very loose, with bleeding from the gingival sulcus.

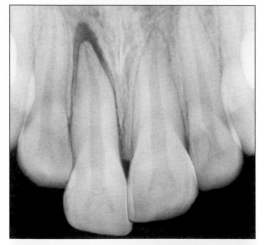

RADIOGRAPHIC APPEARANCE
The tooth appears dislocated, with the apical part of the socket empty.

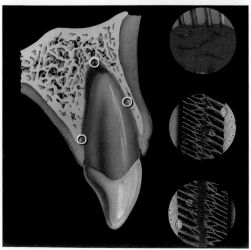

BIOLOGIC CONSIDERATIONS AND TREATMENT PRINCIPLES
The impact results in almost total disruption of the PDL attachment as well as rupture of the apical neurovascular bundle, causing excessive mobility of the tooth and pulpal infarction. The disruption of the neurovascular supply is reflected in negative pulpal sensibility. Healing implies reorganization and re-establishment of the continuity of the PDL fibers as well as pulpal revascularization and reinnervation.[91]

The treatment principle implies repositioning of the tooth in order to facilitate PDL healing. Furthermore, when pulpal revascularization is possible (open or half-open apices), optimal repositioning will facilitate this process, as well as ensure vitality of Hertwig's epithelial root sheath and continued root development. The tooth is splinted to maintain the tooth in an anatomically correct position during the initial healing process and prevent re-extrusion.

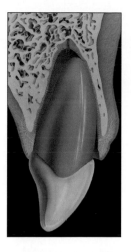
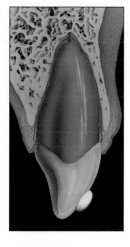

TREATMENT

The extruded tooth should be repositioned gently using axial finger pressure on the incisal edge. Local anesthesia is usually not needed. When the tooth is fully repositioned, check occlusion. Use a nonrigid splint (see page 56). Take a radiograph to control tooth position, and recall the patient after 2–3 weeks and take a new radiograph. If there is no sign of hard tissue changes (i.e. root resorption, bone loss), remove the splint. In cases of teeth with open apices, follow-up including radiographic examination and sensibility testing for extended periods is indicated to diagnose healing complications (primarily pulp necrosis). In cases of teeth with closed apices, the likelihood of revascularization is minimal. Therefore, root canal therapy can be initiated just prior to splint removal. However, an exception to this practice is made for patients where continuous radiographic and pulp testing can be maintained to verify pulpal healing or necrosis.[91-99]

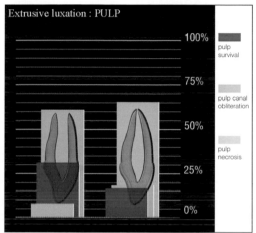

EXPECTED OUTCOME: PULP

In teeth with open apices, pulp canal obliteration is a relatively frequent finding, while pulp necrosis is rare. In teeth with closed apices, the situation is reversed.[90,91]

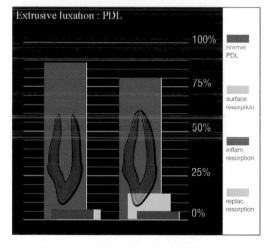

EXPECTED OUTCOME: PDL

Root resorption is rare; and then primarily surface resorption. However, inflammatory resorption can be seen in all stages of root development in association with pulp necrosis.[90,91]

NOTES

Lateral Luxation

OBJECTIVES
1 Differentiate type of luxation injury.
2 Identify injured tissues involved.
3 Define objectives of acute treatment.
4 Estimate frequency and type of possible complications.

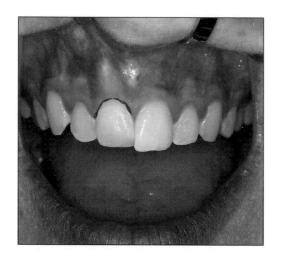

DEFINITION AND CLINICAL APPEARANCE

This trauma implies lateral eccentric displacement of the tooth in its socket; and is accompanied by comminution or fracture of the alveolar bone plate(s).

The tooth appears displaced in its socket, usually in a palatal direction. The tooth is immobile due to its locked position in the socket, and there is a high ankylotic percussion tone. There may or may not be bleeding from the gingival sulcus. The root apex can be palpated in the sulcus area.

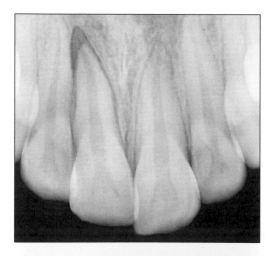

RADIOGRAPHIC APPEARANCE

A steep (occlusal) or eccentric radiographic exposure is necessary to disclose displacement. The tooth appears displaced, with the apical or lateral part of the socket empty.

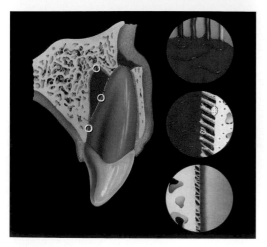

BIOLOGIC CONSIDERATIONS AND TREATMENT PRINCIPLES

The injury is very similar to extrusive luxation. However, it is further complicated by the presence of a fracture of the labial bone plate as well as a compression zone in the cervical area palatally.[100–102]

The treatment principles implies repositioning to facilitate pulpal and periodontal healing; and the tooth should be splinted during the healing period due to marked remodeling processes.

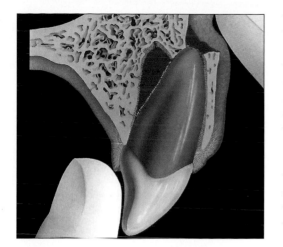

TREATMENT

The displaced tooth is usually locked firmly in its new position. Repositioning requires disengagement of the tooth from its bony lock. Adequate regional anesthesia (infraorbital regional block) is necessary, as repositioning is a painful procedure. The tooth can be repositioned using forceps or digitally, with pressure in an incisal direction over the apex, whereby the tooth is first slightly extruded to disengage the apex and then repositioned in an apical direction. After repositioning, occlusion should be checked and a radiograph taken to verify correct repositioning. The tooth should be splinted for a minimum of 3–4 weeks with a nonrigid splint. A clinical and radiographic control should then be performed. If these controls show no sign of marginal or periradicular breakdown, the splint can be removed. If any of these signs are present, splinting should be maintained for another 3–4 weeks, as the tooth can be very loose at this stage of healing due to transient breakdown of the PDL.

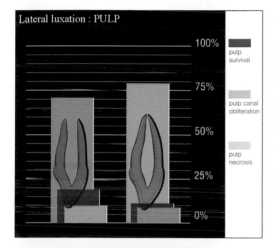

EXPECTED OUTCOME: PULP

In teeth with open apices, observation including radiographic examination and pulp testing is indicated for extended periods in order to diagnose healing complications. In teeth with closed apices, the likelihood of revascularization is minimal. Therefore, root canal therapy can be initiated just prior to splint removal. However, an exception to this practice is made for patients where continuous radiographic and pulp testing can be maintained to assure healing (pulp canal obliteration and/or positive response to sensibility testing) or verify pulp necrosis (periapical lesion or symptoms of pulpitis).[100]

In teeth with open apices pulp canal obliteration is a relatively frequent finding, while pulp necrosis is rare. In teeth with closed apices the situation is reversed.[102]

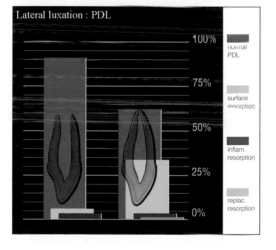

EXPECTED OUTCOME: PDL

Due to compression of the PDL, both inflammatory and replacement resorption (however rare) may occur. Surface resorption is very frequent and usually located apically.[102]

NOTES

Intrusive Luxation

OBJECTIVES

1 Differentiate type of luxation injury.
2 Identify injured tissues involved.
3 Define objectives of acute treatment.
4 Estimate frequency and type of complications.

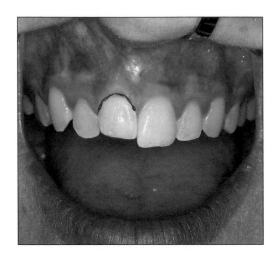

DEFINITION AND CLINICAL APPEARANCE

In this type of luxation the tooth is forced into the socket and locked in position in bone.

Clinically the crown of the tooth appears shortened. There is bleeding from the gingiva. The percussion tone is high and metallic.

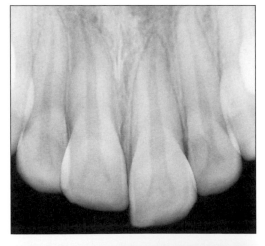

RADIOGRAPHIC APPEARANCE

The tooth appears dislocated in an apical direction with partial disappearance of the periodontal ligament space. This is especially evident cervically. However, the radiographic appearance is not always diagnostic. A high ankylotic percussion tone is usually the pathognomonic feature for diagnosis.

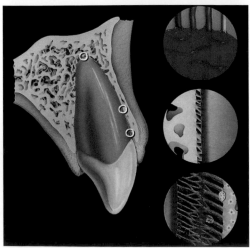

BIOLOGIC CONSIDERATIONS AND TREATMENT PRINCIPLES

Intrusion represents a very complex wound, involving disruption of the marginal gingival seal, contusion of the alveolar bone, disruption of PDL fibers, cementum and disruption of the neurovascular supply to the pulp. Such an injury, which involves contusion of all components of the dentoalveolar complex implies severely compromised healing (see page 11). Optimal PDL healing is dependent on the presence of large noninjured areas of PDL, which is usually not the case after intrusion. Bone will, therefore, often replace the PDL and result in ankylosis (see page 13).[103–109]

At present, the value of acute repositioning of the intruded tooth is uncertain. Spontaneous or guided re-eruption has been found to lead to healing in approximately half of the cases. However, spontaneous re-eruption can normally only be expected to occur in cases with incomplete root formation.

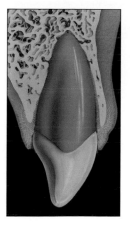
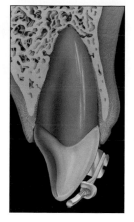

TREATMENT

In teeth with **open apices**. Using infiltration or regional anesthesia, the tooth is grasped with forceps and slightly loosened to release it from its locked position in bone and is then left to re-erupt. Alternatively, orthodontic extrusion can be employed to ensure repositioning of the tooth within 3 weeks after injury, so that interceptive endodontic therapy can be initiated should pulp necrosis and/or inflammatory resorption occur.

In teeth with **closed apices**. In these cases, spontaneous re-eruption is unreliable. Orthodontic extrusion is the treatment of choice. If the tooth has been fully intruded, partial repositioning is necessary to permit bonding of a bracket. Extrusion should be complete within 3 weeks after injury. Prophylactic extirpation of the pulp should then be performed. A close follow-up is indicated, as multiple complications can occur due to the profound PDL and pulpal injuries.

SURGICAL REPOSITIONING

Surgical repositioning appears to give satisfactory healing results up to the age of 12 years. Beyond this age, orthodontic extrusion should be used.[109] In case of surgical repositioning, it is important that the lacerated gingiva is well adapted and sutured around the neck of the tooth. A flexible splint is placed and maintained for 4–8 weeks.

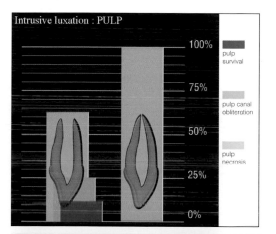

EXPECTED OUTCOME: PULP

Complete healing (revascularization and reinnervation) can only be expected in teeth with incomplete root formation. With increased stages of root development (closed apices), pulp necrosis is especially frequent.[104,105] The most significant prognostic factor appears to be the stage of root development at the time of injury.

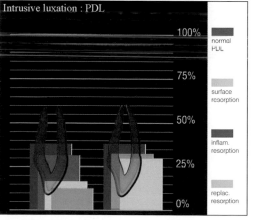

EXPECTED OUTCOME: PDL

External surface, inflammatory and replacement resorption are very frequent findings, especially in teeth with completed root development.[104,105] It should be noted that severe healing complications can be seen as late as 5–10 years after trauma.

NOTES

Avulsion

OBJECTIVES

1 Identify the tissues involved.
2 Provide emergency treatment.
3 Describe type of healing complications.
4 Select treatment options, based on root development and severity of injury.

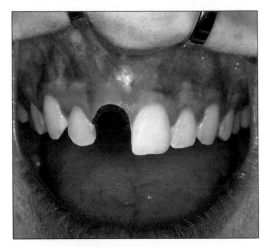

DEFINITION AND CLINICAL APPEARANCE

In this trauma, the tooth is displaced **totally out** of its socket. Clinically the socket is found empty or filled with a coagulum.

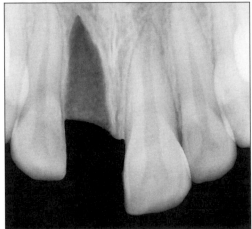

RADIOGRAPHIC APPEARANCE

The socket is empty; fracture lines in the socket may be present.

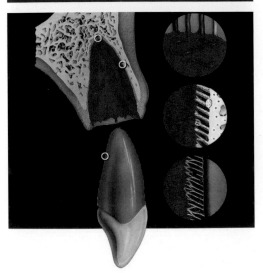

BIOLOGIC CONSIDERATIONS AND TREATMENT PRINCIPLES

Immediately after injury, the PDL and pulp in the avulsed tooth begin to suffer ischemic injury, which is soon aggravated by drying, exposure to bacteria or chemical irritants. These events can kill PDL and pulpal cells even after a short extra-alveolar period.[110–126] Treatment outcome is strongly dependent on the length of the dry extra-alveolar period and storage media.[112–118] If the extra-alveolar period is less than 1 hour, complete or partial PDL healing is possible. However, total PDL death can be expected after more than 1 hour of drying; and progressive root resorption will be the result.[115] In these cases, the indication for replantation should be considered. Thus, in cases of young individuals, where considerable alveolar growth has to take place (i.e. 7–13 years of age), replantation is generally not indicated due to ankylosis and subsequent inter-ference with alveolar growth. In older individuals, where limited alveolar growth is to be expected, replantation can be performed.

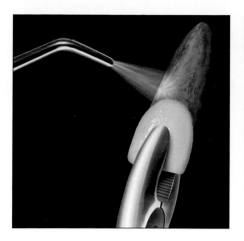
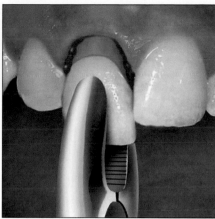
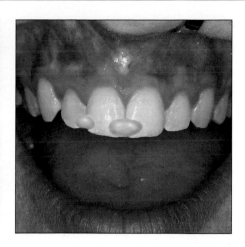

TREATMENT

Replantation of an avulsed tooth preferably should be done at the site of injury in order to minimize extra-alveolar time. In these cases, the tooth should be immediately replanted in its socket or, if obviously contaminated, rinsed for 10 seconds in cold running tap water. The patient should then seek an emergency service or dental office for further treatment, including splinting and antibiotic prophylaxis.

If immediate replantation is not possible, the avulsed tooth should be stored in milk or in the mouth in the oral vestibule. Recently, special storage media have been developed which offer excellent protection to the PDL (e.g. Viaspan® or other media).[127]

Tooth replantation which is performed in a dental office or emergency setting should consist of the following procedures:
Assess extra-alveolar period and storage medium. The following conditions will question or exclude replantation: age of the patient; extensive carious destruction of the tooth; extensive loss of marginal periodontal support; medically compromising situations (e.g. infectious endocarditis, immunosuppressive treatment).

If immediate replantation is indicated, the following steps should be carried out:
1 Rinse the tooth surface carefully with a flow of physiological saline from a syringe. All obvious contaminants should be removed. Persistent contamination should be removed with gauze sponges saturated in saline.
2 Flush the socket coagulum with saline.
3 Replant the tooth slowly with gentle digital pressure. The tooth must not be forced into place. If any resistance is met, the tooth should be removed and stored in saline while the socket is examined for any bony fractures.
4 Splint the tooth with a semi-rigid splint (see page 56).
5 Antibiotic coverage should be given (e.g. penicillin 1000 mg immediately, thereafter 500 mg four times daily for 4 days).[110]
6 Tetanus prophylaxis is assessed according to the immunization status of the patient.

In the extended extra-alveolar periods in adults, an alternative replantation procedure is possible, whereby the replantation becomes "implantation", in that the root surface is treated with a fluoride solution to make the root surface partially osteoclast resistant and thereby protract the replacement process of any later ankylosis.[128]

The steps in this procedure are the following:
1 Remove the necrotic PDL from the avulsed tooth with scalers and/or pumice.
2 Extirpate the pulp.
3 Place the tooth in a 2% NaF solution (pH = 5.5) for 20 minutes.
4 Root fill the tooth extraorally with gutta percha and sealer.
5 Rinse the root surface for 2 minutes with saline.
6 Replant the tooth after removing the coagulum from the socket.
7 Splint the tooth for 6 weeks.

In cases of extensive extra-alveolar dry storage, a doubling of the tooth survival time can be expected.[128]

FOLLOW-UP

The splint is removed after 1 week (immediate replantation). If pulpal revascularization is not to be expected (teeth with closed apices), the pulp is extirpated prior to splint removal and calcium hydroxide is placed in the root canal as an interim dressing. Completion of the root canal treatment is described on page 60. In all cases, a radiographic control should be made after 2 or 3 weeks. At this time, signs of inflammatory resorption may be present, which will dictate pulpal extirpation, even in teeth with incomplete root formation.[113,129] Further radiographic and clinical controls should be made after 2 and 6 months, 1, 2 and 5 years at which time ankylosis, if it is going to occur, can usually be demonstrated.[115,130] Pulpal and periodontal healing have been found to be dependent on three factors:[112–115]

• length of extra-alveolar storage

• extra-alveolar storage medium

• stage of root development.

In the graphs on pages 50 and 51, the survival rates of pulp, periodontal ligament and tooth survival are presented as they relate to the above-mentioned factors.

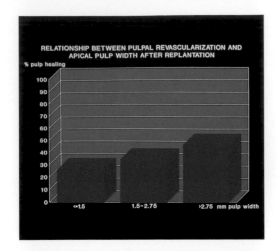

EXPECTED OUTCOME: PULP
Healing appears related to the width of the apical foramen.[113]

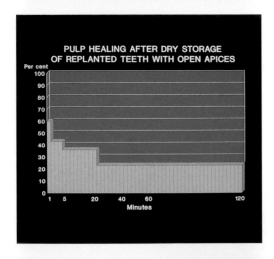

EXPECTED OUTCOME: PULP
Healing appears related to the length of the pulp.[113]

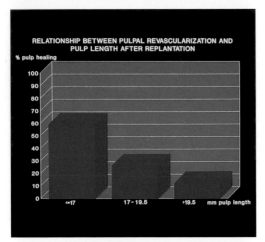

EXPECTED OUTCOME: PULP
Healing appears related to the length of the dry extra-alveolar period.[113]

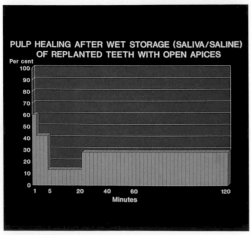

EXPECTED OUTCOME: PULP
Healing appears related to length of the wet extra-alveolar period (saliva/saline).[113]

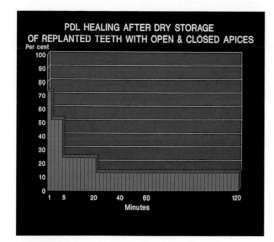

EXPECTED OUTCOME: PDL

Healing appears related to the length of the dry extra-alveolar period for teeth with incomplete and complete root formation.[115]

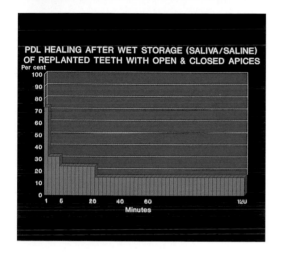

EXPECTED OUTCOME: PDL

Healing appears related to the length of the wet extra-alveolar period for teeth with incomplete and complete root formation (saliva/saline).[115]

ENDODONTIC CONSIDERATIONS

Due to the associated pulp and PDL injury, the risk of root resorption is eminent. Consequently, the following endodontic treatment rules are suggested based on present experimental and clinical studies,[110–131] as well as recommended guidelines.[119,120]

TEETH WITH CLOSED APICES

Pulp revascularization is not likely to occur; and as a prophylactic measure against development of root resorption the pulp should be extirpated 7–10 days after replantation.[110,113] Calcium hydroxide is placed in the root canal and the tooth should be permanently root filled with gutta percha and a sealer after 2–4 weeks.

TEETH WITH OPEN APICES

Pulp revascularization is possible. Pulp necrosis is usually evident after 2–4 weeks and presents with periapical rarefaction with or without signs of inflammatory root resorption.[110,113] As soon as the diagnosis pulp necrosis has been made, the pulp should be extirpated and the root canal biomechanically cleansed and medicated with calcium hydroxide. This technique is described on page 60.

Injuries to the Primary Dentition

OBJECTIVES
1 Recognize the various trauma entities in the primary dentition.
2 Recognize the risk of subsequent trauma to the permanent dentition.
3 Determine treatment options aimed at reducing the risk of disturbances in development of the permanent.
4 Determine risk profile for primary tooth trauma which presents a significant risk for the permanent dentition successors.

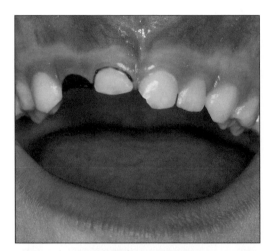

DEFINITION AND CLINICAL APPEARANCE

These traumas result in loss of tooth substance or displacement of the primary tooth.

The clinical appearance of traumas in the primary dentition is similar to that in the permanent dentition. This figure demonstrates an avulsion (right lateral incisor) and intrusion (right central incisor) and an uncomplicated crown fracture (left central incisor).

RADIOGRAPHIC APPEARANCE

Similar to findings in the permanent dentition. However, an important goal in the radiographic examination is to determine whether the primary tooth has invaded the developing follicle.

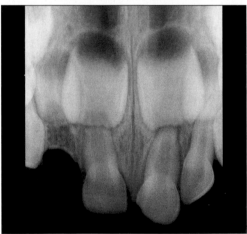

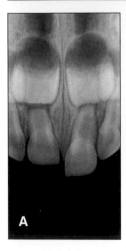
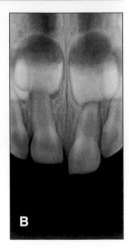

RADIOGRAPHIC APPEARANCE: WITH OR WITHOUT INVASION OF THE FOLLICLE

A foreshortened image of the luxated tooth implies that the primary root apex has been forced facially, away from the follicle (A).[132,133] An elongated image suggests displacement in the opposite direction, and thus a risk for the developing tooth (B). The developing teeth should appear symmetric. If the distance between the incisal edge and the mineralization front of the developing tooth is less on the injured side than on the noninjured side (B), there is a significant risk that the intruded primary tooth has dislocated the developing permanent tooth germ. This finding indicates immediate removal of the primary tooth.

BIOLOGIC CONSIDERATIONS

The very close proximity of the developing permanent successors to the apices of the primary teeth makes the transmission of trauma due to luxation injuries a very likely event.[134]

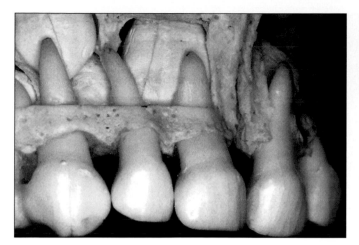

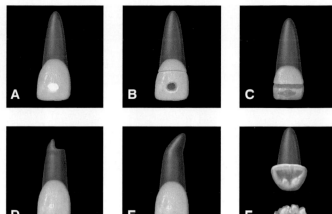

Moreover, inflammation related to pulpal complications of the displaced tooth may add further injury.[132] In fact, approximately one-half of all primary tooth injuries result in more or less severe disturbances in permanent tooth development. These disturbances range from mineralization disturbances to complete malformation of the tooth germ, as illustrated: (A) white or yellow enamel opacity, (B) yellow–brown enamel opacity with or without hypoplasia, (C) yellow–brown enamel opacity with circumferential hypoplasia, (D) partial arrest of root formation, (E) root dilaceration, (F) root angulation and odontoma-like malformation.

TREATMENT PRINCIPLES

The primary goal is to optimize periodontal and pulpal healing in the primary dentition provided that no further injury is transmitted to the developing permanent successor.[132]

Recent animal studies indicate that similar pulpal and periodontal healing responses to acute dental traumas are found in both dentitions.[132] Concerning transmission of trauma to the developing successor, the major effect seems to originate from the initial trauma, with little effect from repositioning or extraction of the displaced primary tooth. One exception, however, is when the primary tooth is intruded directly into the follicle and immediate extraction of the primary tooth appears to be the treatment of choice.[132]

Periapical infection may occur due to an infected pulp necrosis in the primary tooth. This indicates extraction of the primary tooth to avoid a known long-term effect of inflammation on mineralization of the permanent tooth germ.[132]

TREATMENT

Treatment is related to the type of trauma.

Crown fractures

Uncomplicated fractures are treated by smoothing of sharp edges. Teeth with exposed pulps are usually extracted due to lack of patient cooperation. However, pulp capping or pulpotomy may be performed.

Crown-root fractures

These teeth should be extracted.

Root fractures

Displaced coronal fragments can be repositioned. However, splinting is generally neither possible and nor necessary. Should

pulp necrosis occur, the coronal fragment is extracted, while the apical fragment is left to be resorbed physiologically. The permanent tooth will then erupt normally.[132]

Concussion and subluxation

Observation.

Extrusion

Extraction or careful repositioning.

Lateral luxation

Most laterally luxated teeth are displaced with the crowns in a palatal direction. This implies that the apex is displaced away from the permanent tooth germ. If there is no occlusal interference, the tooth is allowed to reposition spontaneously.

Intrusion

Due to the labial curvature of the apex, most intruded teeth are displaced through the labial bone plate. These teeth can, therefore, be left to re-erupt spontaneously. A few teeth are intruded directly into the developing tooth germ and should be removed.

Avulsion

A radiographic examination is essential to ensure that the missing tooth is not intruded. Avulsed primary teeth should not be replanted.[132]

Fracture of the alveolar process

The fragment is repositioned and splinted if possible (see page 36).

FOLLOW-UP

Close controls are necessary to diagnose healing complications. These are primarily pulpal complications related to infected pulp necrosis following luxation injuries; and are related to the type of luxation.[133,135] Postoperative controls should be performed 4, 8 and 26 weeks and 1 year after injury. In cases of complicated trauma (intrusion and avulsions), a further radiographic control is indicated just before eruption of the permanent successor to register any disturbances in tooth development or eruption.

EXPECTED OUTCOME

The long-term prognosis should define the fate of the injured primary tooth and the permanent successor. The risk of pulp necrosis in the primary dentition appears to be related to the type of luxation injury.[133] The risk of disturbances in the permanent dentition appears also to be related to the type of luxation injury (see following pages).[134–141]

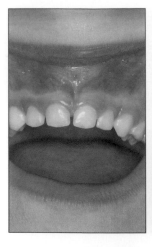 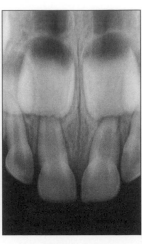 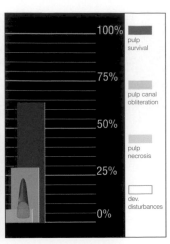

CONCUSSION

Pulp healing is frequent.[133,135]

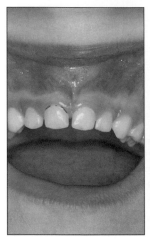 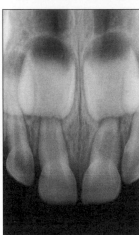 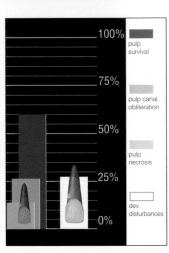

SUBLUXATION

Pulp healing is frequent. Complications in the permanent dentition are relatively rare and usually consist of enamel hypoplasias.[133,135]

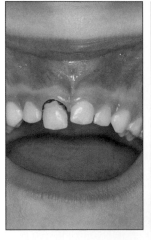 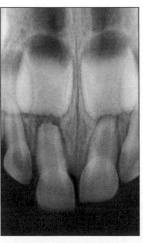 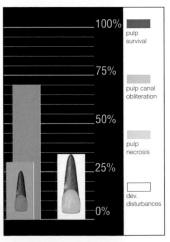

EXTRUSION

Pulp healing is dependent upon stage of root development. There is moderate risk of complications in the permanent dentition.[133,135]

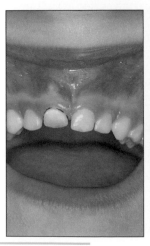 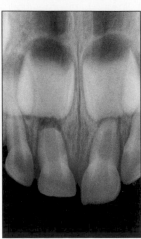 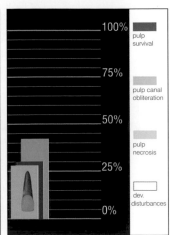

LATERAL LUXATION

Pulp healing is dependent on the stage of root development.[133]

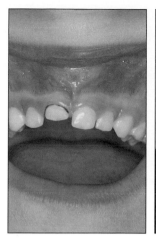 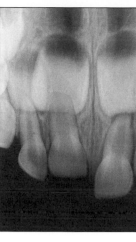 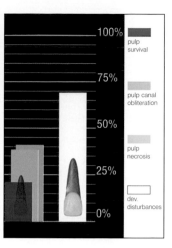

INTRUSION

Pulp necrosis is frequent, as are complications in the permanent dentition.[133,135]

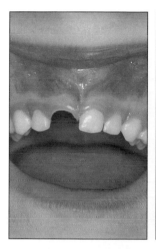 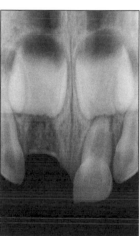 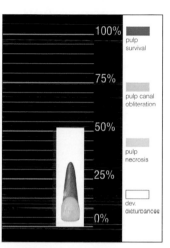

AVULSION

Complications in the permanent dentition are frequent.[135]

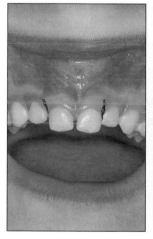 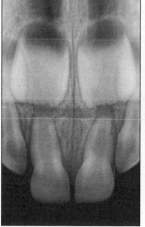 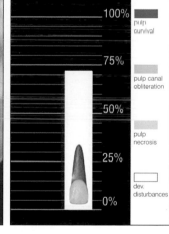

FRACTURE OF THE ALVEOLAR PROCESS

Complications in the permanent dentition are frequent.[135]

NOTES

_____

_____

_____

_____

_____

Splinting

OBJECTIVES 1 Describe application of two types of semirigid splints.
2 Describe removal of a semirigid splint.

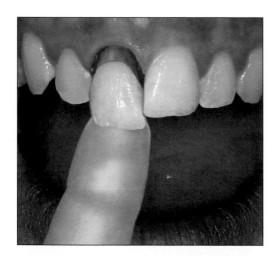

REPOSITIONING

The injured tooth is repositioned and occlusion checked. A radiograph is taken to ensure adequate repositioning. Semi-rigid splinting (in contrast to rigid splinting) has been found to be essential in creating optimal healing conditions for the injured periodontal ligament as well as the pulp.[142–150] See also page 15.

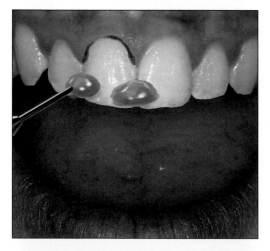

ETCHING ENAMEL

The incisal one-third of the labial aspect of enamel on the injured and adjacent teeth is acid-etched (30 seconds) with phosphoric acid gel.

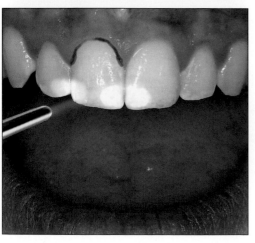

RINSING AND DRYING ENAMEL

The etchant is removed with a 20-second water spray and the enamel dried with a stream of compressed air; the etched enamel has a matte, chalky appearance. The teeth are isolated with gauze sponges labially and palatally. Hemostasis can be achieved by compressing these sponges with firm finger pressure.

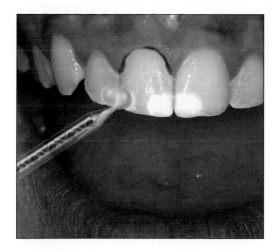

APPLYING SPLINTING MATERIAL

The splinting material is applied in a thin layer. If a temporary bridge material (e.g. Protemp®, Luxatemp®, Isotemp®, Provipond®) is used, a semi-rigid splint is created. If composite is used, rigid splinting is the result (see page 15). During polymerization of the splinting material, have the patient occlude to ensure correct repositioning of the tooth. Keep the splint away from the gingiva to permit optimal oral hygiene.

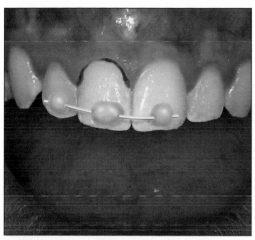

GLASS FIBER/KEVLAR® FIBER/RIBBOND® FIBER/ORTHODONTIC WIRE SPLINT

Semi-rigid splinting alternatives include the use of the above-mentioned materials. It is important that the reinforcing wires are placed inside the composite or temporary bridge material for labial bonding of the injured and adjacent teeth.

Bonded orthodontic brackets can also be used. This form of splinting has the advantage in multiple tooth injuries that the various splinting periods can be respected without removing the splint.

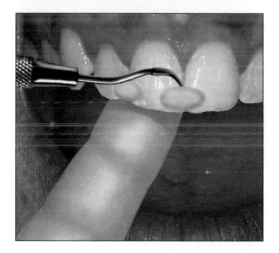

REMOVING THE SPLINT

At the end of the fixation period, the splint is removed with either a scaler or a fissure bur. The enamel is then lightly polished to re-establish a smooth surface.

NOTES

_____

_____

_____

_____

_____

_____

Endodontic Implications of Dental Trauma

OBJECTIVES

1 Recognize differences in caries and trauma-related pulp pathosis.
2 Define treatment goals.
3 Determine the effects of bacteria on healing events after trauma.
4 Recognize how resorption processes may interfere with the endodontic procedures.
5 Recognize the endodontic problems of exposed pulps in teeth with open and closed apices with vital pulps.
6 Recognize the endodontic problems of necrotic pulps in teeth with root fractures.
7 Recognize the endodontic problems of teeth with associated external root resorption.

PULP AND PERIODONTAL LIGAMENT PATHOLOGY FOLLOWING DENTAL CARIES AND DENTAL TRAUMA

There appears to be major differences in etiology and pathogenesis of pulp and pathology related to caries progression and dental trauma.[151] The main therapeutic problem following caries-related infected pulp necrosis appears to be control of bacteria in the pulp canal. However, due to mature root formation, obturation is usually an uncomplicated procedure. In cases of trauma-related pulp necrosis (see page 11) and the frequently open apex, problems in root canal obturation are often encountered. Furthermore, infection-related external root resorption (see page 12) cannot be arrested without proper sterilization of the root canal and dentinal tubules. Finally, due to its remodeling character, ankylosis can expose dentinal tubules, resulting in direct or indirect exposure of the potentially contaminated root canal content.

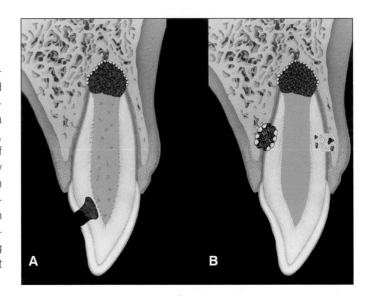

IMPLICATIONS OF PULP NECROSIS AND DEVELOPING ROOT FORMATION: TREATMENT OBJECTIVES

An open apex represents a major obstacle in sterilizing and later obturating the root canal. Experimental and clinical studies have shown that bacteria are usually limited to the necrotic pulp and dentinal tubules. Removal of necrotic pulp tissue and sterilization of the root canal will lead to healing processes, which in most cases imply closure of the apical area by a hard tissue barrier formed by cementoblasts. In rare cases where the Hertwig's epithelial root sheath has survived, dentin and cementum may be formed (apexogenesis). Due to the frequently weakened structure of the immature root, treatment approaches should be selected which do not further weaken the tooth (i.e. extensive filing or extensive chemical treatment of the canal (e.g. prolonged placement of calcium hydroxide)), which could lead to spontaneous fracture.

IMPLICATIONS OF INFECTION-RELATED ROOT RESORPTION

The presence of infection-related root resorption cavities on the root surface represents a significant threat to the prognosis of the endodontic procedure. Unless all bacteria are permanently removed or inactivated in the root canal as well as the dentinal tubules, resorption may progress. Whereas, if bacteria are removed or inactivated, healing will take place with a new periodontal ligament or an ankylosis (in case of extensive resorption cavities).

IMPLICATION OF ANKYLOSIS-RELATED RESORPTION

Due to the inherently progressive nature of the ankylosis process (see page 12), where dentinal tubules may be exposed by osteoclastic activity, effective root canal obturation is essential. Furthermore, a bacteria tight seal must be created at the entrance of the root canal. Unless these steps are taken, a slowly progressive resorption may change to a rapidly invading infection-related resorption.

TIME RELATION OF VARIOUS PROPERTIES OF CALCIUM HYDROXIDE

For decades, calcium hydroxide has been known to be a very effective medication in the treatment of pulpal and periodontal complications following injury. This is primarily related to simultaneous sterilization of tissue and the capacity to invite hard tissue healing. Knowledge about the time relationship of these effects is necessary for its proper use. Calcium hydroxide is known to have a strong proteolytic effect.[152] Thus, most pulp remnants will be totally dissolved within 1 week. However, the same proteolytic effect apparently also affects the circumpulpal dentin, resulting over time (months) in weakening.[153] This is possibly the explanation for the occurrence of cervical fractures in more than half of the endodontically treated teeth with immature root formation.[154] The use of calcium hydroxide should therefore be limited to a few weeks.

Pulp necrosis with or without infection-related resorption: completed root formation

After pulp extirpation, calcium hydroxide is used as an interim root canal dressing to desinfect the root canal and dentinal tubules, to dissolve necrotic pulp remnants and to arrest osteoclastic activity on the root surface. After 2 weeks, the root canal space is obturated with gutta percha and a sealer. It is

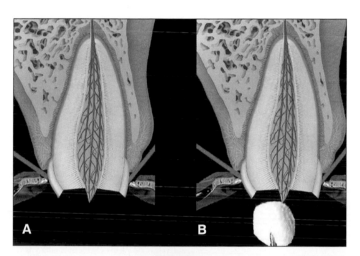

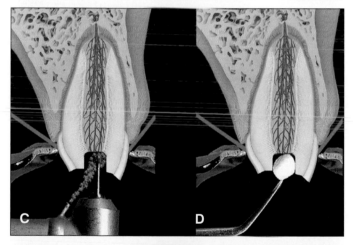

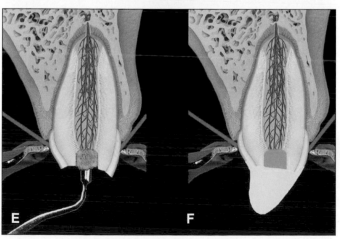

important to create a bacteria tight seal in the cervical region in order to prevent reactivation of resorption processes or periapical inflammation.

TREATMENT OF TRAUMATIC DENTAL INJURIES USING MINERAL TRIOXIDE AGGREGATE

Mineral trioxide aggregate (MTA; ProRoot MTA, Root Canal Repair Material Dentsply Tulsa Dental, Tulsa, OK, USA) has been shown to be a very useful dental material for the treatment of many conditions, including traumatic dental injuries. The material is currently used in vital pulp therapy, as apical plugs in teeth with open apices, and to provide a barrier at the site of root fractures when the coronal pulp in such teeth must be extirpated and replaced with a filling material.[155–162]

PULP CAPPING AND PULPOTOMY

Pulp capping and pulpotomy are procedures aimed at protecting the vital pulp from bacterial invasion and, in young teeth, allow for continued root development. Calcium hydroxide has been the most commonly used agent, in combination with restorative materials, for achieving these goals. MTA has several advantages over calcium hydroxide: it provides protection against bacterial penetration, does not disintegrate over time, and after setting provides a hard surface against which other dental materials can be placed.[157–160] Pulp capping with calcium hydroxide is described on page 30. The use of MTA in connection with pulpotomy is described in the following.

(A) Isolate the tooth with rubber dam after administering local anesthesia.

(B) Disinfect the exposed dentin and pulp with either sodium hypochlorite or Peridex[®].

(C) Remove pulp and surrounding dentin to a depth of 2 mm from the level of exposure, using a round diamond bur and water or saline spray.

(D) Place a saline-moistened cotton pellet onto the pulpal wound until bleeding has ceased, or nearly so. Slight hemorrhage does not affect placement of MTA.

(E) A mixture of MTA and saline or water can now be placed into the prepared cavity against the pulpal wound and fill the entire cavity.

(F) After setting (4–6 hours), a restoration can be placed to restore the tooth or bond the fractured crown fragment. While setting, the MTA serves as a temporary restoration. Thus, the patient should be instructed to avoid chewing or biting, as the material initially is quite soft.

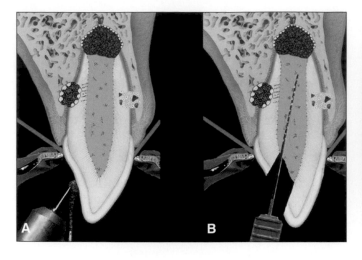 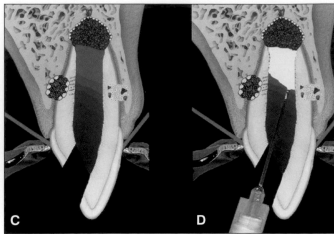

TREATMENT OF PULP NECROSIS IN IMMATURE TEETH

In situations where the pulp becomes necrotic before the root is fully developed, the apical opening is too large to create a stop for the root canal filling. Apexification procedures using calcium hydroxide have been performed with reasonable success.[151] The disadvantage in using calcium hydroxide for apexification is that it can take many months to obtain enough of an apical barrier to allow placement of a root canal filling.[151] Additionally, it now appears that long-term use can weaken dentin and result in cervical fracture on slight impact or even physiological use.[153,154]

By using MTA as a physical barrier apically, a root canal filling can be placed immediately without waiting for a biological response.[155,156,161,162] Also, by minimizing exposure of root dentin to calcium hydroxide, there is less desiccation of dentin. The technique is as follows.

(A) The tooth is isolated with rubber dam, the crown disinfected, and an access cavity to the root canal prepared.

(B) Extirpation of necrotic pulp tissue is done to a level apically where fresh bleeding from healthy tissue is encountered. This can be anywhere from several millimeters from the apex to flush with the apical foramen.

(C) Root canal preparation in developing teeth requires a conservative approach, so as to preserve as much root dentin as possible. Hence minimal canal shaping is appropriate.

(D) Disinfection of the root canal with sodium hypochlorite is followed by short-term (approximately 2–4 weeks) interim dressing with calcium hydroxide. The use of calcium hydroxide allows acceptable disinfection of the root canal system and provides a dry root canal, free of seepage of apical exudates. The coronal access opening must be sealed with a dependable temporary restoration.

(E) At the next visit, the calcium hydroxide is removed and the canal is thoroughly irrigated with saline or sodium hypochlorite to obtain a debris-free canal. Small increments of the MTA/water mixture are introduced into the canal and gently condensed. Length can be controlled using a rubber stopper on a plugger. No harm is done, however, with slight overfilling.

(F) When properly condensed, the apical MTA plug should be at least 4 mm thick. The entire canal can be filled with MTA (to the cervical level), or the coronal part of the canal can later be filled with gutta percha and sealer.

(G) To allow setting, a moistened (water) cotton pellet is placed in the access cavity, which is then sealed with a temporary filling material. Once set (usually within 4–6 hours), the canal can be conventionally filled.

(H) The temporary material and cotton pellet are removed, the apical plug is checked for setting hardness; it should not be vigorously probed, as the material can break. The canal is then irrigated, dried and filled, followed by a bonded coronal composite restoration.

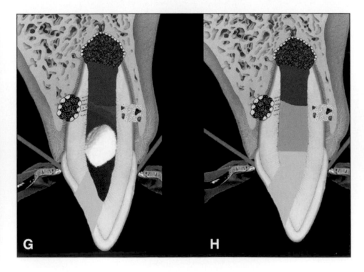

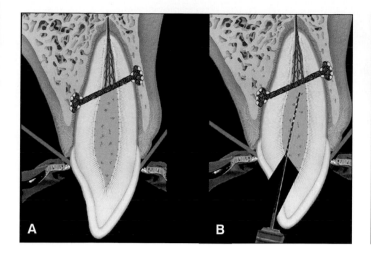

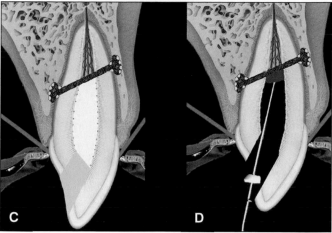

TREATMENT OF ROOT FRACTURES

Intra-alveolar root fractures will typically heal if properly managed, and if so, endodontic intervention is not necessary.

(A) In some instances, however, the coronal pulp undergoes necrosis, due to lack of revascularization, and requires root canal treatment (see page 34).

(B) The recommended procedure has been to isolate the tooth with rubber dam, extirpate the necrotic coronal pulp, and clean and prepare the canal to the fracture site. This was then followed by placement of calcium hydroxide to obtain a hard tissue barrier at the level of fracture.[151] As in teeth with open apices, calcium hydroxide has been quite successful in inducing a hard tissue

barrier; but usually requires several months. Moreover, desiccation of dentin may also be a disadvantage in the use of calcium hydroxide.

(C) In a manner similar to the open apex situation, MTA can be used to create a physical barrier at the fracture site. The technique is the same as described above, the only difference being the level of placement.

(D) As the distance from the fracture site to the coronal orifice may be quite short, it is advisable to fill the entire coronal root canal until the cervical level with MTA. As in the above-mentioned procedures, setting of MTA should be confirmed before final restoration with dentin-bonded composite.

NOTES

Tooth Survival Following Various Trauma Entities in the Permanent Dentition

OBJECTIVE   1   Identify low-, medium- and high-risk trauma with respect to tooth survival.

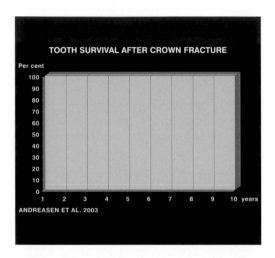

CROWN FRACTURES

The following graphs represent a recent study on the long-term prognosis of various trauma entities.[163] Irrespective of presence or absence of pulp exposure, crown fractures have an optimal long-term prognosis.[163]

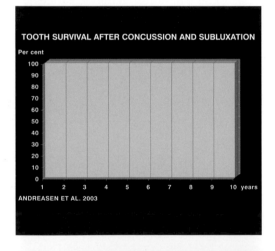

CONCUSSION AND SUBLUXATION

Both trauma entities have optimal long-term tooth survival.[163]

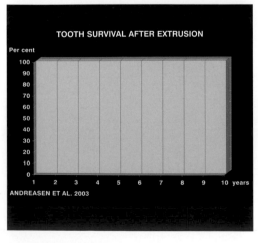

EXTRUSION

Tooth survival is to a certain degree related to tooth development at time of injury, but the chance of long-term survival is very good.[163]

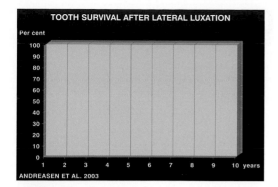

LATERAL LUXATION

Tooth survival is to a certain degree related to tooth development at time of injury, but the chance of long-term survival is very good.[163]

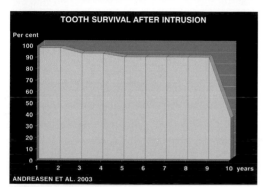

INTRUSION

Tooth survival is strongly related to tooth development at time of injury. The leading cause of failure is progression of inflammatory and/or ankylosis-related resorption. Due to generally poor long-term survival, treatment alternatives (e.g. orthodontic space closure, transplantation of premolars, implants or fixed prosthetics) should be considered, especially if replacement or infection-related resorption occurs.[163]

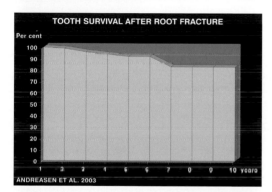

ROOT FRACTURES

Long-term survival is related to the type of healing. This graph illustrates that both healing with hard tissue (HT), connective tissue (CT), and successfully treated pulp necrosis (GT) have good long-term prognoses.[163]

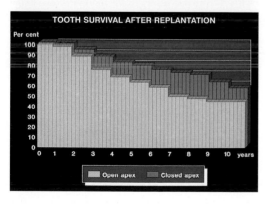

AVULSION AND REPLANTATION

The most significant factors determining long-term survival appear to be storage time and storage media[163] due to the obvious large variations in the combination of these two factors, it is not possible in this context to present survival scenarios for all possible combinations.

In a larger long-term clinical study of 400 replanted teeth, roughly half of the replanted teeth had 15-years' survival, with a slight preference to teeth with immature root formation.

NOTES

_____

_____

_____

_____

_____

_____

Information for the Patient About Dental Trauma

OBJECTIVE   **1**   This section is an example of the information that you can prepare for patients that have suffered a traumatic dental injury.

When teeth or jaws have been injured, many questions arise. Can the injury be treated? How much time is needed? What does it cost? Is treatment covered by insurance or public agencies? We will try to answer these questions here. Because this section covers many different questions, the dentist who has treated you will mark the sections that apply to your injury.

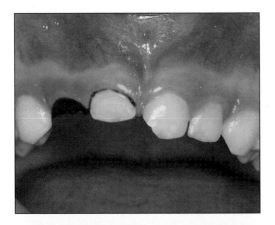

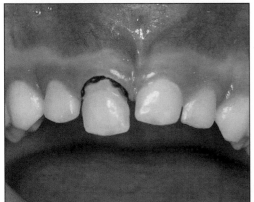

PRIMARY TOOTH INJURIES

Most often, there is just loosening of the primary (milk) tooth; but In some cases, the tooth is forced into the jaw. An X-ray will be taken to register the extent of injury and to determine whether the permanent tooth bud – which lies just under the primary tooth root – has also been affected.

If this is the case, it may be necessary to remove the primary tooth to ensure normal development of the permanent tooth. If the primary tooth is not too close to the permanent tooth bud, we can just wait for the loosened primary tooth to tighten up, which usually happens within a few weeks. In this healing period, it's very important that your child avoid hard foods; but that doesn't mean a liquid diet. The use of a pacifier should be limited as much as possible.

Primary teeth that are forced into the jaw will usually grow out again within 2–4 months. In rare cases, an acute infection of the root can develop, which will cause pain, severe swelling and pain, fever, severe redness around the injured tooth. It is very important that this infection is treated by your dentist immediately, so that it doesn't spread to the permanent tooth.

Injured primary teeth should always be checked every 1–2 months and 1 year after injury to make sure that there has been no injury to the permanent tooth bud. In all circumstances, such an injury should be reported to your insurance company, because some cases result in damage to the permanent teeth that require treatment at a later date.

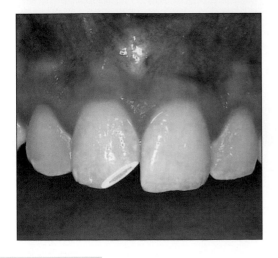

FRACTURE OF PERMANENT TEETH

Fractures of the crown of the tooth can vary in extent. If only a corner of the enamel is involved, usually only slight grinding is necessary.

If the fracture has exposed dentin, it is necessary to restore the tooth either with a tooth-colored plastic material or porcelain. If the tooth chip has been found, it can be reattached with a special glue. This can be done at the time of injury or at a later date; but it's important that the chip is kept moist, by storing it in a glass of water. The water should be changed daily.

If the nerve has been exposed, it must be covered with a special material that lets the hole into the nerve be closed with new dentin. This usually takes 2–3 months. However, the final restoration can be made over this dressing either in the form of tooth-colored plastic or reattachment of the tooth chip. Porcelain veneers or crowns can be made later, once the patient is adult.

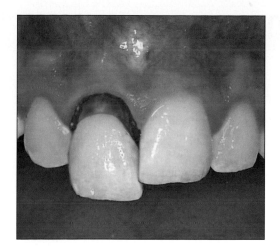

LOOSENING OF THE TOOTH OR FRACTURE OF THE ROOT OF A PERMANENT TOOTH

In some cases,, loosening of the tooth means that the nerve dies. In these cases, the dead nerve must be removed and replaced by a root filling. In rare cases this can lead to discoloration of the crown of the tooth. Tooth bleaching or a porcelain crown can correct this problem.

FRACTURE OF THE JAW

In these cases it is often necessary to place splints on the teeth in the upper and lower jaw and then bind the lower jaw to the upper. This is done to ensure that the fracture heals in the right position. Normally the jaws must be bound together for 3–6 weeks, depending on the fracture's severity. A special liquid diet is prescribed during this period.

DIET

In some cases, when the teeth have been loosened, a splint will not be applied. Instead, a soft diet will be prescribed for the first 14 days, to protect the injured teeth. A soft diet means no hard foods; but not necessarily a liquid diet.

ORAL HYGIENE

Careful tooth brushing should be performed as soon as possible after injury. Meticulous cleansing of the teeth and gums is a prerequisite for rapid healing. Daily oral hygiene includes the following:

1 After every meal rinse your mouth thoroughly with Hibitane Dental® (this can be purchased at your pharmacy).
2 Careful tooth brushing after every meal, with a soft tooth-brush, working from the gums to the teeth in the upper and lower jaws. In difficult areas, a solo toothbrush can be used (can be purchased at your pharmacy).
3 After tooth brushing, make sure that splints and teeth are completely clean.

In some cases, it is necessary to take X-rays 3 or 6 weeks and 1 year after injury to control healing. X-rays are taken to diagnose possible late healing complications, such as infection of the root or jaw. Your dentist will make these appointments.

POLICE REPORT

If the injury can be expected to lead to a court trial (e.g. an assault or a road-traffic accident), it is important that the police are notified as soon after injury as possible as to the cause of the injury. This report could be used in a later trial.

NOTES

_____
_____
_____
_____
_____
_____

Information for the Public About Dental Trauma

OBJECTIVES
1. Inform the community about the importance of preventing and treating dental trauma.
2. Describe specific ways, suitable for different age groups, in which dental trauma can be prevented.
3. Recommend appropriate emergency measures to be taken immediately following dental trauma.

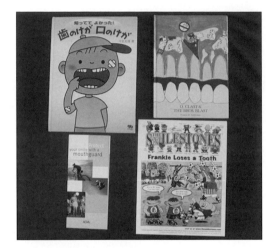

DEVELOPING PUBLIC DENTAL TRAUMA AWARENESS

Because so little public health education has addressed issues related to dental health, the proposed campaign must be focused so as to present its message clearly, making the population aware of its role in saving teeth in case of an accident.[164–173] Target groups in this effort would be those groups exposed to a high risk of accident: children, adolescents and the adult population should be included in this task.[164] This could be done via picture storybooks,[165,173] manuals, information included in natural science textbooks, posters, brochures, television programs, television and radio talk shows, the local press and, most recently, multimedia.

Even when the use of mouthguards, helmets and facemasks has been widely recommended, there is insufficient evidence of their effectiveness in changing the behavior of players in reducing the frequency of sports-related injuries to the head, face and mouth.[167] Injury prevention campaigns addressing the need for protective devices in sports and bicycling can increase awareness and use. This can rapidly be achieved through legislation or regulation.[164]

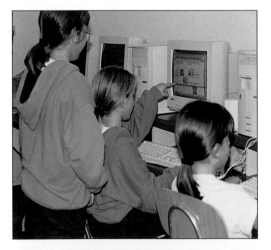

INTERNET USE IN TRAUMA EDUCATION AND PREVENTION

The Internet is a useful communication tool. It is an effective form of spreading knowledge, accessible at very low cost to many potential users.[168–173] One of its weaknesses is that the information provided does not always have scientific references. It would be desirable that scientific information could be provided for dentists through the web system at university sites. Although many web addresses have a commercial interest, information is provided in a direct and entertaining manner to the general public.

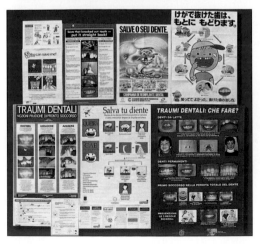

TRAUMA BROCHURES AND POSTERS

Many countries have made special efforts to reach the public with educational material, in the form of brochures, posters and dental trauma information campaigns. These countries include Australia, Argentina, Brazil, Chile, Denmark, Finland, France, Israel, Italy, Japan, Norway and Sweden. Furthermore, the International Association of Dental Traumatology has developed and collected brochures and posters which can be obtained at the following address: Dr. M.T. Flores, Department of Pediatric Dentistry, Faculty of Dentistry, University of Valparaiso, Valparaiso, Chile.

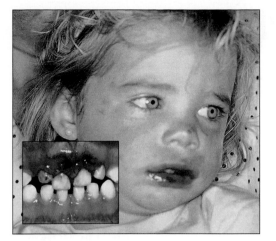

FIRST-AID AND TREATMENT OF TRAUMA TO PRIMARY TEETH

Recommendations for the public when responding to dental trauma in young children should include the following measures:

- Wash the wound with plenty of running water. Generally, dental trauma includes injuries to the adjacent soft tissue.
- Stop bleeding by compressing the injured area with gauze or cotton wool for 5 minutes.
- Seek emergency treatment from a pediatric dentist.

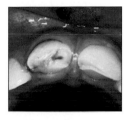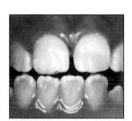

FIRST-AID AND TREATMENT FOR TRAUMA TO PERMANENT TEETH

Tooth fractures (broken teeth), luxations (loosened or displaced teeth) and avulsions (complete loss of the tooth) are the most frequent injuries to the permanent teeth which could have an improved outcome if the public were well informed about appropriate first-aid measures.

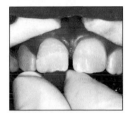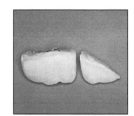

FIRST-AID FOR A CROWN FRACTURE

With a crown fracture, the broken piece of tooth may be repositioned using dental adhesives and composite resins.

- Find the tooth fragment and place it in a glass of water.
- Seek dental treatment immediately.

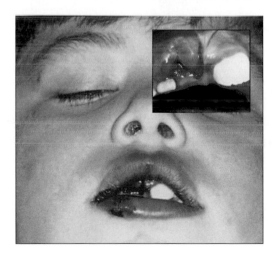

FIRST-AID FOR AN AVULSED TOOTH

Often a permanent tooth can be saved through appropriate first-aid and immediate treatment.

- Find the tooth and pick it up by the crown.
- If the tooth is dirty, wash briefly (10 seconds) under cold running water and reposition it.
- If this is not possible, place the tooth in a glass of milk. The tooth can also be transported in the mouth, keeping it between the teeth and the cheek.
- Seek emergency dental treatment immediately.

NOTES

_____

_____

_____

_____

_____

_____

Prevention of Traumatic Dental Injuries

OBJECTIVES
1. Identify medium- and high-risk sports.
2. Describe preventive measures.
3. Describe effects of prevention measures.

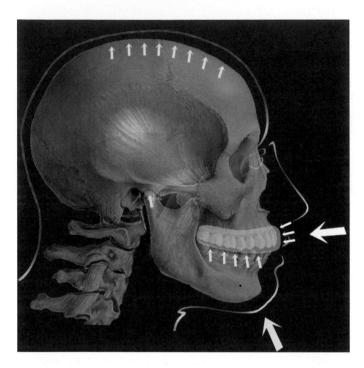

MECHANISM OF MOUTHGUARD PROTECTION

All sports activities are connected with a certain risk of orofacial injuries due to falls, collisions and contact with hard surfaces. Contact sports, such as ice hockey, football, handball, soccer and basketball, with their strong risk of collisions at high speed, are especially prone to result in dental and other injuries.[174–177] Clinical and experimental evidence suggest that mouthguards can help to distribute energy from impact, and thereby reduce the risk of severe injury.[179–182,184]

The mechanism of mouthguard protection varies depending on the energy and direction of impact. If the impact hits the base of the mandible, the cushioning effect of the elastic mouthguard material between the mandible and the maxilla reduces the force of impact occlusally, as well as preventing crown and crown-root fractures. In the condylar region, the forces of impact are also reduced, whereby the risk of brain concussion is minimized.[179] With a frontal impact, the impact force is reduced again due to the material's elasticity and by distribution of forces over a greater area.[180,181] Whether this implies that the risk of fracture is replaced by risk of tooth luxations remains to be examined. In several types of sports the use of mouthguards seems to reduce the risk of dental injuries.[182]

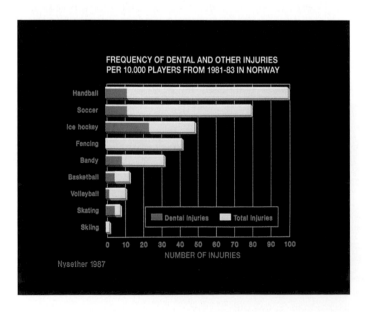

FREQUENCY OF DENTAL AND OTHER INJURIES PER 10.000 PLAYERS FROM 1981-83 IN NORWAY

Nysether 1987

DENTAL AND OTHER INJURIES RELATED TO VARIOUS SPORTS

Based on insurance records, a very precise documentation of dental and other injuries exists from Norway.[183] In this report, ice hockey was found to be associated with the highest risks. Sports-related injuries are usually very costly.[178]

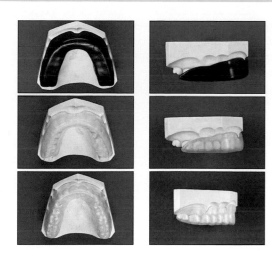

VARIOUS TYPES OF MOUTH PROTECTORS

- Stock variety protectors are of latex rubber or polyvinyl chloride, usually made in three sizes and supposed to be universally fitting; the advantage being their low cost. However, they have been found to impede both speech and breathing, as they can only be kept in place by occlusion. There is no evidence that they can redistribute forces of impact.

- Mouth-formed protectors: varieties are fitted from a manufactured kit consisting of a fairly rigid outer shell and a soft resilient heat-cured or self-cured lining. These protectors have the advantage of a better fit, while still being quite inexpensive.

- Custom-made protectors are individually processed by a dentist or dental technician on plaster models of the athlete's dental arches. The pressure-laminated variety seems to afford most protection.[184] These protectors, while significantly more expensive than stock or mouth-formed protectors, have been found to be acceptable and comfortable for most athletes.

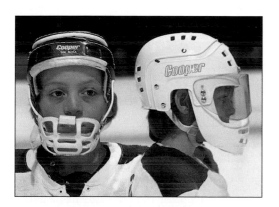

FACE MASKS

Face masks are used extensively in ice hockey.[179] They have been found to be very effective in protecting players from orofacial injuries since the use of helmet, facemasks, and mouthguards became mandatory in organized contact sports, such as football and ice hockey in the USA and northern countries.[185]

In a recent study of ice hockey players, it was shown that both full and partial facial protection reduces injuries to the eyes and face from 159 to 23 injuries per 1000 player-game hours.[174]

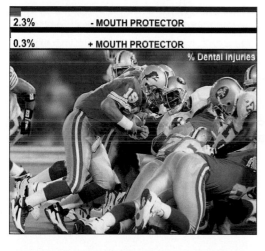

EFFECT OF MOUTHGUARDS AND FACE MASK PROTECTION IN AMERICAN FOOTBALL

Roberts studied the incidence of dental injuries in American football over a period of 14 years in Wisconsin, USA. During this period, a dramatic reduction in the annual incidence was seen – first with the introduction of facemasks and later by the addition of mouthguards.[185] Similar figures have been reported in Finland.[186.]

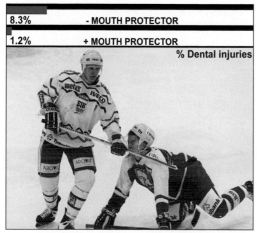

EFFECT OF MOUTHGUARD PROTECTION IN ICE HOCKEY

Ice hockey is the contact sport, which is associated with the greatest risk of orofacial injury. Thus, a study of professional Canadian ice hockey players showed that 62% had lost one or more incisors.[177] The use of mouthguards in ice hockey in Canada has been shown to decrease the annual rate of dental injuries from 8.3% to 1.2%.[177]

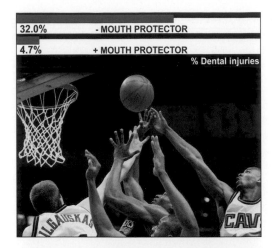

EFFECT OF MOUTHGUARD PROTECTION IN BASKETBALL

A North American study reported a dramatic decrease in the frequency of orofacial injuries in players using mouthguards in the 1986–7 varsity basketball season.[187] About two-thirds of the injuries recorded consisted of lacerations and bruises. A recent prospective study led to the conclusion that custom-fitted mouthguards did not significantly affect rates of brain concussions or oral soft tissue injuries, but could significantly reduce the morbidity and expense resulting from dental injuries in men's college basketball.[188]

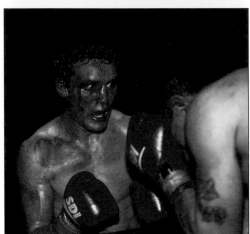

EFFECT OF MOUTHGUARDS IN BOXING

Boxing was probably one of the first sports activities where the need for mouthguards was recognized. In the boxing world championship held in Cuba in 1975, no oral injuries were found after examination of 250 boxers, all of them wearing mouthguards.[189]

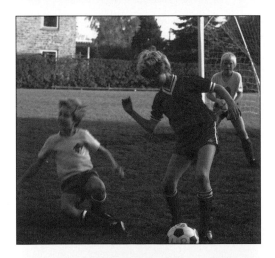

EFFECT OF MOUTHGUARDS IN SOCCER

Soccer is probably the most widespread sports activity in the world today. Being a contact sport, it is known to involve a high risk of injuries especially to extremities, but also oral injuries are frequent. This risk is especially high for goalkeepers and forwards; and is also strongly related to the more experienced teams.[183]

Studies from the USA and Japan reported oral injuries incidences of 28% and 32%, respectively, among high school soccer players in a 2-year season.[175,176] In both studies, almost none of the players used mouthguards.

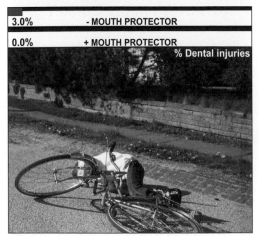

EFFECT OF HELMET PROTECTION IN BICYCLING

Head injuries are very frequent in bicycle accidents. In Victoria, Australia mandatory helmet protection was introduced in 1990. After 1 year of helmet law, there was a 48% reduction of head injuries.[190]

Oral and maxillofacial injuries are frequent in bicycle accidents in children aged younger than 15 years. However, current helmets offer no protection against injuries to the lower part of the face including dental injuries,[191–193] whereas mouthguards offer protection against dental injuries.[182]

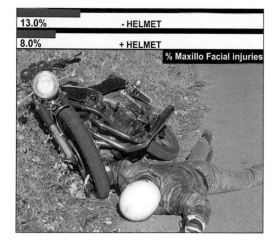

13.0% - HELMET
8.0% + HELMET
% Maxillo Facial injuries

EFFECT OF HELMET PROTECTION IN MOTORCYCLE-RELATED INJURIES

Motorcycle injuries are a major source of fatal and nonfatal head trauma in the USA. The use of helmets reduces maxillofacial injuries by up to 50%.[194,195]

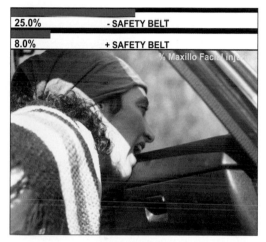

25.0% - SAFETY BELT
8.0% + SAFETY BELT
% Maxillo Facial injuries

EFFECT OF SAFETY BELTS IN MOTOR VEHICLE-RELATED INJURIES

Motor vehicle-related injuries are known to lead to frequent dental and maxillofacial injuries. Front-seat passengers are particularly at risk, due to collision with the front panel or steering wheel. In a study from the USA, it was shown that the use of safety belts reduced the frequency of facial injuries by 30%.[196]

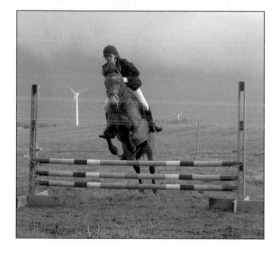

EFFECT OF HELMET PROTECTION IN HORSEBACK RIDING

Horseback riding is known not only to be a sporting activity with a very high incidence of injury, but also of severe injuries, sometimes with a fatal outcome. These injuries are usually caused by falls from the horse, collision with branches when riding in forests or by horse kicks when standing behind the horse. The use of helmets, especially with a strap protecting the chin can prevent some of these injuries. However, no statistics exist on the extent of prevention.

NOTES

Appendix 1

Emergency record for acute dental trauma

| Patient's name |
| Birth date |

| Date of examination: | Referred by: |
| Time of examination: | Referring diagnosis: |

General medical history: any serious illness? yes no
If yes, explain.
Any allergy? yes no
If yes, explain.
Have you been vaccinated against tetanus? yes no
If yes, when.

Previous dental injuries: yes no
If yes,
  When?
  Which teeth were injured?
  Treatment given and by whom?

Present dental injury:
  Date: Time:
  Where?
  How?

Have you had or have now *headache?* yes no

Have you had or have now *nausea?* yes no

Have you had or have now *vomiting?* yes no

Were you *unconscious* at the time of injury? yes no
If yes, for how long (minutes)?
Can you *remember* what happened before, yes no
during or after the accident?

Is there pain from *cold air?* yes no
If yes, *which teeth?*

Is there pain or tenderness from *occlusion?* yes no
If yes, *which teeth?*

Constant pain? yes no
If yes, *which teeth?*

Treatment elsewhere? yes no
If yes, *what treatment?*

Emergency record for acute dental trauma

After *avulsion*, the following information is needed:
Where were the teeth found (dirt, asphalt, floor, etc.)?
When were the teeth found?
Were the teeth *dirty?*
How were the teeth *stored?*
Were the teeth *rinsed* and *with what* prior to replantation?
When were the teeth replanted?
Was *tetanus antitoxoid* given?
Were *antibiotics* given?
  Antibiotic?
  Dosage?

Objective examination

Is the patient's general condition affected?	yes	no

If yes, *pulse*
    blood pressure
    pupillary reflex
    cerebral condition

Objective findings beyond the head and neck?	yes	no

If yes, *type* and *location*

Objective findings within the head and neck?	yes	no

If yes, *type* and *location*

Objective examination – Extraoral findings (contd.)

Bleeding from nose, or rhinitis	yes	no
Bleeding from ext. auditory canal	yes	no
Double vision or limited eye movement	yes	no
Palpable signs of fracture of facial skeleton	yes	no

If yes, *location of fracture*

Objective examination – Intraoral findings

Lesions of the *oral mucosa*	yes	no

If yes, *type* and *location*

Gingival lesion	yes	no

If yes, *type* and *location*

Tooth fracture	yes	no

If yes, *type* and *location*

Alveolar fracture	yes	no

If yes, *type* and *location*

Supplemental information:

General condition of the dentition

Caries	poor	fair	good
Periodontal status	poor	fair	good
Horizontal occlusal relationship	undr bite	over jet	norm
Vertical occlusal relationship	deep	open	norm

Emergency record for acute dental trauma

Radiographic findings
Tooth dislocation
Root fracture
Bone fracture
Pulp canal obliteration
Root resorption

Photographic registration   [yes] [no]

Diagnoses (check appropriate boxes and designate tooth no. or indicate correct anatomical region)

☐ Infraction   ☐ Skin abrasion
☐ Complicated crown fracture   ☐ Skin laceration
☐ Uncomplicated crown fracture   ☐ Skin contusion

☐ Complicated crown-root fracture   ☐ Mucosal abrasion
☐ Uncomplicated crown-root fracture   ☐ Mucosal laceration
                                      ☐ Mucosal contusion

☐ Root Fracture
☐ Alveolar fracture
☐ Mandibular fracture   ☐ Gingival abrasion
☐ Maxillary fracture   ☐ Gingival laceration
                                      ☐ Gingival contusion

☐ Concussion   *Supplementary remarks:*
☐ Subluxation
☐ Extrusion
☐ Lateral luxation
☐ Intrusion
☐ Exarticulation

Treatment plan
At time of injury: *Final therapy:*
Repositioning (time finished)
Fixation (time finished)
Pulpal therapy (time finished)
Dentinal coverage (time finished)

*Chart re-*read by examining dentist   [yes] [no]

Appendix 2

Clinical examination form for the time of injury and follow-up examinations

		Tooth no.		12		11		21		22	
T **I** **M** **E** **O** **F** **I** **N** **J** **U** **R** **Y**		Date									

		Tooth color
		  normal
		  yellow
		  red
		  grey
		  crown restoration									

		Displacement (mm)
		  intruded
		  extruded
		  protruded
		  retruded									

		Loosening (0-3)									
		Tenderness to percussion (+/-)									
		Pulp test (value)									
		Ankylosis tone (+/-)									
		Occlusal contact (+/-)									
C **O** **N** **T** **R** **O** **L**		Fistula (+/-)									
		Gingivitis (+/-)									
		Gingival retraction (mm)									
		Abnormal pocketing (+/-)									

Each column represents an examination of a given tooth. The first column for each tooth gives the values from the time of injury. *Only* the parameters listed in the top half of the form ("Time of injury") are to be recorded at the time of injury. The information from this examination as well as the information collected on the emergency record are used to determine the final diagnoses for the injured teeth. Those parameters *and* the last four (fistula, gingivitis, gingival retraction, abnormal pocketing) are to be registered at all follow-up controls.

Appendix 3

Clinical and radiographic findings with the various luxation types

Findings	Concussion	Subluxation	Extrusion	Lateral Luxation	Intrusion
Clinical					
Abnormal mobility	–	+	+	-(+)	-(+)
Tenderness to percussion	+	+(-)*	+/-	-(+)	-(+)
Percussion sound**	normal	dull	dull	metallic	metallic
Response to pulp testing	+/-	+/-	-(+)	-(+)	-(+)
Clinical dislocation	–	–	+	+	+
Radiographic dislocation	–	–	+	+	+

* A sign in parentheses indicates a finding of rare occurrence.

** Teeth with incomplete root formation and teeth with marginal or periapical inflammatory lesions will also elicit a dull percussion sound.

Bibliography

EPIDEMIOLOGY OF TRAUMA DENTAL INJURIES

1. **Andreasen JO, Andreasen FM.** Classification, etiology and epidemiology of traumatic dental injuries. In: Andreasen JO, Andreasen FM eds. *Textbook and Color Atlas of Traumatic Injuries to the Teeth*, 3rd edn. Copenhagen: Munksgaard, 1993: 151–177.

   Since the 1993 edition the following epidemiologic studies have been published.

2. **Caliskan MK, Turkun M.** Clinical investigation of traumatic injuries of permanent incisiors in Izmir, Turkey. *Endod Dent Traumatol* 1995; **11**: 210–213.

3. **Carvalho JC, Vinker F, Ceclerck D.** Malocclusion, dental injuries and dental anomalies in the primary dentition of Belgian children. *Int J Paediatr Dent* 1998; **8**: 137–141.

4. **Chen YL, Tsai TP, See LC.** Survey of incisor trauma in second grade students of central Taiwan. *Changgeng Yi Xue Zhi* 1999; **22**: 212–219.

5. **Hamdan MA, Rock WP.** A study comparing the prevalence and distribution of traumatic dental injuries among 10–12-year-old children in an urban and in a rural area of Jordan. *Int J Paediatr Dent* 1995; **5**: 237–241.

6. **Marcenes W, al Beiruti N, Tayfour D, Issa S.** Epidemiology of traumatic injuries to the permanent incisor of 9–12-year-old schoolchildren in Damascus, Syria. *Endod Dent Traumatol* 1999; **15**: 117–123.

7. **Marcenes W, Zabot NE, Traebert J.** Socio-economic correlates of traumatic injuries to the permanent incisors in schoolchildren aged 12 years in Blimenau, Brazil. *Dent Traumatol* 2001; **17**: 222–226.

8. **Mestrinho HD, Bezerra AC, Carvalho JC.** Traumatic dental injuries in Brazilian pre-school children. *Braz Dent J* 1998; **9**: 101–104.

9. **Petti S, Cairella G, Tarsitani G.** Childhood obesity: a risk factor for traumatic injuries to anterior teeth. *Endod Den Traumatol* 1997; **13**: 285–288.

10. **Otuyemi OD, Segun-Ojo IO, Adegboye AA.** Traumatic anterior dental injuries in Nigerian preschool children. *East Afr Med J* 1996; **73**: 604–606.

11. **Rai SB, Munshi AK.** Traumatic injuries to the anterior teeth among South Kanar school children – a prevalence study. *J Indian Soc Pedod Prev Dent* 1998; **16**: 44–51.

12. **Glendor U, Halling A, Andersson L, Eilert-Petersson E.** Incidence of traumatic tooth injuries in children and adolescent in country of Västmanland, Sweden. *Swed Dent J* 1996; **20**: 15–28

13. **Crona-Larson G, Noren JG.** Luxation injuries to permanent teeth – a retrospective study of aetiological factors. *Endod Dent Traumatol* 1985; **5**: 176–179.

NATURE AND CONSEQUENCES OF TRAUMA

14. **Gottrup F, Andreasen JO.** Wound healing subsequent to injury. In: Andreasen JO, Andreasen FM eds. *Textbook and Color Atlas of Traumatic Injuries to the Teeth*, 3rd edn. Copenhagen: Munksgaard, 1993: 13–76.

15. **Andreasen JO, Torabinejad M, Finkelman RD.** Response of oral tissue to trauma and inflammation and mediators of hard tissue resorption. In: Andreasen JO, Andreasen FM eds. *Textbook and Color Atlas of Traumatic Injuries to the Teeth*, 3rd edn. Copenhagen: Munksgaard, 1993: 77–133.

16. **Andreasen JO.** Experimental dental traumatology: development of a model for external root resorption. *Endod Dent Traumatol* 1987; **3**: 269–287.

17. **Andreasen JO.** Review of root resorption systems and models. Etiology of root resorption and the homeostatic mechanisms of the periodontal ligament. In: Davidovitch Z ed. *The Biological Mechanisms of Tooth Eruption and Root Resorption*. Birmingham: EBSCO Media; 1988: 9–21.

18. **Andreasen JO.** Summary of root resorption. In Davidovitch Z ed. *The Biological Mechanisms of Tooth Eruption and Tooth Resorption*. Birmingham: EBSCO Media, 1988: 399–400.

19. **Andreasen JO, Andreasen FM.** Root resorption following traumatic dental injuries. *Proc Fiin Dent Soc* 1991; **88**: 95–114.

20. **Hammarström L, Pierce A, Blomlöf L, Feiglin B, Lindskog S.** Tooth avulsion and replantation – a review. *Endod Dent Traumatol* 1986; **2**: 1–8.

21. **Hammarström L, Lindskog S.** General morphological aspects of resorption of teeth and alveolar bone. *Int Endodont J* 1985; **18**: 93–108.

22. **Pierce AM, Lindskog S, Hammarström L.** Osteoclasts: structure and funktion. *Electron Microsc Rev* 1991; **4**: 1–45.

23. **Cvek M, Cleaton-Jones P, Austin J, Kling M, Lownie J, Fatti P.** Effect of topical application of doxycycline on pulp revascularization and periodontal healing in reimplanted monkey incisors. *Endod Dent Traumatol* 1990; **6**: 170–176.

24. **Pierce AM.** Experimental basis for the management of dental resorption. *Endod Dent Traumatol* 1989; **5**: 255–265.

25. **Hammarström L, Blomlöf L, Feiglin B, Lindskog S.** Replantation of teeth and antibiotic treatment. *Endod Dent Traumatol* 1986; **2**: 51–57.

26. **Sae-Lim V, Wang CY, Choi GW, Trope M.** The effect of systemic tetracycline on resorption of dried replanted dogs' teeth. *Endod Dent Traumatol* 1998; **14**: 127–132.

27. **Cvek M, Cleaton-Jones P, Austin J, King M, Lownie J, Fatti P.** Pulp revascularization in reimplanted immature monkey

incisors – predictability and the effect of antibiotic systemic prophylaxis. *Endod Dent Traumatol* 1990; **6**: 157–169.

28. **Yanpiset K, Trope M.** Pulp revascularization of replanted immature dog teeth after different treatment methods. *Endod Dent Traumatol* 2000; **16**: 211–217.

CLASSIFICATION OF DENTAL INJURIES

29. **Andreasen JO, Andreasen FM.** Classification, etiology and epidemiology of traumatic dental injuries. In: Andreasen JO, Andreasen FM eds. *Textbook and Color Atlas of Traumatic Injuries to the Teeth*, 3rd edn. Copenhagen: Munksgaard Publishers, 1993: 151–177.

30. **Application of the International Classification of Diseases to Dentistry and Stomatology.** IDC-DA, 3rd edn. Geneva: WHO, 1995.

EXAMINATION AND DIAGNOSIS

31. **Andreasen FM, Andreasen JO.** Examination and diagnosis of dental injuries. In: Andreasen JO, Andreasen FM eds. *Textbook and Color Atlas of Traumatic Injuries to the Teeth*, 3rd edn. Copenhagen: Munksgaard Publishers, 1993: 106–216.

32. **Andreasen FM, Andreasen JO.** Diagnosis of luxation injuries. The importance of standardized clinical, radiographic and photographic techniques in clinical investigations. *Endod Dent Traumatol* 1985; **1**: 160–169.

33. **Bakland LK, Andreasen JO.** Examination of the dentally traumatized patient. *Calif Dent Ass J* 1996; **24**: 35–44.

DIAGNOSIS OF PULP HEALING COMPLICATIONS

34. **Andreasen JO.** Response of oral tissue to trauma. In: Andreasen JO, Andreasen FM eds. *Textbook and Color Atlas of Traumatic Injuries to the Teeth*, 3rd edn. Copenhagen: Munksgaard, 1993: 77–112.

35. **Andreasen FM, Vestergaard Pedersen B.** Prognosis of luxated

permanent teeth – the development of pulp necrosis. *Endod Dent Traumatol* 1985; **1**: 207–220.

36. **Andreasen FM, Yu Z, Thomsen BL.** Relationship between pulp dimensions and development of pulp necrosis after luxation injuries in the permanent dentition. *Endod Dent Traumatol* 1986; **2**: 90–98.

37. **Andreasen FM, Yu Z, Thomsen ML, Andersen PK.** Occurrence of pulp canal obliteration after luxation injuries in the permanent dentition. *Endod Dent Traumatol* 1987; **3**: 103–115.

38. **Stålhane I.** Permanente tænder med reducerat pulpalumen son följd av olyksfallskada. *Svensk Tandläkar-Tid* 1971; **64**: 311–316.

39. **Jacobsen I, Kerekes K.** Long-term prognosis of traumatized permanent anterior teeth showing calcifying processes in the pulp cavity. *Scand J Dent Res* 1977; **85**: 588–598.

40. **Andreasen FM.** Transient apical breakdown and its relation to color and sensibility changes after luxation injuries to teeth. *Endod Dent Traumatol* 1986; **2**: 9–19.

DIAGNOSIS OF PERIODONTAL HEALING COMPLICATIONS

41. **Andreasen JO, Torabinejad M, Finkelman RD.** Response of oral tissue to trauma and inflammation and mediators of hard tissue resorption. In: Andreasen JO, Andreasen FM eds. *Textbook and Color Atlas of Traumatic Injuries to the Teeth*, 3rd edn. Copenhagen: Munksgaard, 1993: 77–133.

42. **Andreasen JO, Hjørting-Hansen H.** Replantation of teeth. I. Radiographic and clinical study of 110 human teeth replanted after accidental loss. *Acta Odont Scand* 1966; **24**: 263–286.

43. **Andreasen FM, Andreasen JO.** Root resorption following traumatic dental injuries. *Proc Finn Dent Soc* 1992; **88**: 95–114.

44. **Andreasen FM, Andreasen JO.** Resorption and mineralization processes following root fracture of permanent incisors. *Endod Dent Traumatol* 1988; **4**: 202–214.

45. **Andreasen FM, Sewerin I, Mandel U, Andreasen JO.**

Radiographic assessment of simulated root resorption cavities. *Endod Dent Traumatol* 1987; **3**: 21–27.

46. **Andreasen JO, Borum MK, Andreasen FM.** Progression of root resorption after replantation of 400 avulsed human incisors. In: Davidovitch D ed. *The Biological Mechanisms of Tooth Eruption, Resorption and Replacement by Implants*. Boston, MA: Harvard Society for the Advancement of Orthodontics, 1994: 577–582.

TREATMENT PRIORITIES AFTER DENTAL TRAUMA

47. **Andreasen JO, Andreasen FM, Skeie A, Hjørting-Hansen E, Schwartz O.** Effect of treatment delay upon pulp and periodontal healing of traumatic dental injuries – a review article. *Dent Traumatol* 2002; **18**: 1–13.

48. **Cvek M, Andreasen JO, Andreasen FM, Søllner H, Mejare I.** Healing of 445 intra-alveolar root fractures, 2003; study in progress.

49. **Andreasen JO, Andreasen FM.** Intrusion of permanent teeth. Effect of treatment modalities, 2003; study in progress.

CROWN FRACTURE WITHOUT PULP EXPOSURE

50. **Andreasen JO, Andreasen FM.** Crown fractures. In: Andreasen JO, Andreasen FM. *Textbook and Color Atlas of Traumatic Injuries to the Teeth*, 3rd edn. Copenhagen: Munksgaard, 1993: 219–250.

51. **Andreasen FM, Norén JG, Andreasen JO, Engelhardtsen S, Lindh-Strömberg U.** Long-term survival of crown fragment bonding in the treatment of crown fractures. A multicenter clinical study of fragment retention. *Quintessence Int* 1995; **26**: 669–681.

52. **Farik B, Kreiborg S, Andreasen JO.** Adhesive bonding of fragmented anterior teeth. *Endod Dent Traumatol* 1998; **14**: 119–123.

53. **Ravn JJ.** Follow-up study of permanent incisors with enamel cracks as a result of an acute trauma. *Scand J Dent Res* 1981; **89**: 117–123.

54. **Ravn JJ.** Follow-up study of permanent incisors with enamel cracks as a result of an acute trauma. *Scand J Dent Res* 1981; **89**: 213–217.

55. **Ravn JJ.** Follow-up study of permanent incisors with enamel dentin fractures after acute trauma. *Scand J Dent Res* 1981; **89**: 355–365.

56. **Robertson A, Andreasen FM, Andreasen JO, Norén JG.** Long-term prognosis of crown-fractured permanent incisors. The effect of stage of root development and associated luxation injury. *Int J Paediatric Dent* 2000; **10**: 191–199.

57. **Robertson A.** A retrospective evaluation of patients with uncomplicated crown fractures and luxation injuries. *Endod Dent Traumatol* 1998; **14**: 245–256.

58. **Stålhane I, Hedegård B.** Traumatized permanent teeth in children aged 7–15 years. Part II. *Swed Dent J* 1975; **68**: 157–169.

CROWN FRACTURE WITH PULP EXPOSURE

59. **Cvek M.** Endodontic management of traumatized teeth. In: Andreasen JO, Andreasen FM eds. *Textbook and Color Atlas of Traumatic Injuries to the Teeth*, 3rd edn. Copenhagen: Munksgaard, 1993: 517–585.

60. **Ravn JJ.** Follow-up study of permanent incisors with complicated crown fractures after acute trauma. *Scand J Dent Res* 1982; **90**: 363–372.

61. **Cvek M.** A clinical report on partial pulpotomy and capping with calcium hydroxide in permanent incisors with complicated crown fracture. *J Endod* 1978; **4**: 232–237.

62. **Cvek M.** Partial pulpotomy in crown-fractures incisors – results 3 to 15 years after treatment. *Acta Stomatologica Croatica* 1993; **27**: 167–173.

CROWN-ROOT FRACTURE

63. **Andreasen FM, Andreasen JO.** Crown-root fractures. In: Andreasen JO, Andreasen FM eds. *Textbook and Color Atlas of Traumatic Injuries to the Teeth*, 3rd edn. Copenhagen: Munksgaard, 1993: 257–276.

64. **Tegsjö U, Valerius-Olsson H, Olgart K.** Intra-alveolar transplantation of teeth with cervical root fractures. *Swed Dent J* 1978; **2**: 73–82.

65. **Kahnberg K-E, Warfvinge J, Birgersson B.** Intraalveolar transplantation (I). The use of autologous bone transplants in the periapical region. *Int J Oral Surg* 1982; **11**: 372–379.

66. **Kahnberg K-E.** Intraalveolar transplantation of teeth with crown-root fractures. *J Oral Surg* 1985; **43**: 38–42.

67. **Kahnberg K-E.** Surgical extrusion of root fractured teeth – a follow-up study of two surgical methods. *Endod Dent Traumatol* 1988; 45–89.

68. **Warfvinge J, Kahnberg K-E.** Intraalveolar transplantation of teeth. IV. Endodontic considerations. *Swed Dent J* 1989; **13**: 229–233.

ROOT FRACTURE

69. **Andreasen FM, Andreasen JO.** Root fractures In: Andreasen JO, Andreasen FM eds. *Textbook and Color Atlas of Traumatic Injuries to the Teeth*, 3rd edn. Copenhagen: Munksgaard, 1993: 279–311.

70. **Andreasen FM, Andreasen JO, Bayer T.** Prognosis of root fractured permanent incisors – prediction of healing modalities. *Endod Dent Traumatol* 1989; **5**: 11–22.

71. **Andreasen FM, Andreasen JO.** Resorption and mineralization processes following root fracture of permanent incisors. *Endod Dent Traumatol* 1988; **4**: 202–214.

72. **Andreasen FM.** Pulpal healing after luxation injuries and root fracture in the permanent dentition. Thesis, Copenhagen University, 1995. ISBN 87-985537-0-1.

73. **Cvek M.** Treament of non-vital permanent incisors with calcium hydroxide. IV. Periodontal healing and closure of the root canal in the coronal fragment of teeth with intra-alveolar fracture and vital apical fragment. *Odont Revy* 1974; **25**: 239–245.

74. **Birch R, Rock WP.** The incidence of complications following root fracture in permanent anterior teeth. *Br Dent J* 1986; **160**: 119–122.

75. **Cvek M, Andreasen JO, Borum MK.** Healing of 208 intraalveolar root fractures in patients aged 7–17 years. *Dent Traumatol* 2001; **17**: 53–62.

76. **Cvek M, Mejàre I, Andreasen JO.** Healing and prognosis of teeth with intraalveolar fractures involving the cervical part of the root. *Dent Traumatol* 2002; **18**: 57–65.

77. **Majorana A, Pasini S, Bardellini E, Keller E.** Clinical and epidemiological study of traumatic root fractures. *Dent Traumatol* 2001; **18**: 77–80.

78. **Welbury RR, Kinirons MJ, Day P, Gregg TA.** Outcome for root-fractured permanent incisors: a retrospective study. *Pediatric Dentistry* 2002; **24**: 89–102.

79. **Jacobsen I, Zachrisson BU.** Repair characteristics of root fractures in permanent anterior teeth. *Scand J Dent Res* 1975; **83**: 355–364.

80. **Zachrisson BU, Jacobsen I.** Long-term prognosis of 66 permanent anterior teeth with root fracture. *Scand J Dent Res* 1975; **83**: 345–354.

81. **Jacobsen I.** Root fractures in permanent anterior teeth with incomplete formation. *Scand J Dent Res* 1976; **84**: 210–217.

FRACTURE OF THE ALVEOLAR PROCESS

82. **Andreasen JO.** Injuries to the supporting bone. In: Andreasen JO, Andreasen FM eds. *Textbook and Color Atlas of Traumatic Injuries to the Teeth*, 3rd edn. Copenhagen: Munksgaard, 1993: 427–453.

83. **Andreasen JO.** Fractures of the alveolar process of the jaw. A radiographic follow-up study. *Scand J Dent Res* 1970; **78**: 263–272.

84. **Freihofer HPM.** Ergebnisse der Behandlung vom Alveolarforsatzfrakturen. *Schweiz Monatschr Zahnheilk* 1969; **79**: 623–629.

CONCUSSION

85. **Andresen FM, Andreasen JO.** Luxation injuries. In: Andreasen JO, Andreasen FM eds. *Textbook and Color Atlas of Traumatic Injuries to the Teeth*, 3rd edn. Copenhagen: Munksgaard, 1993: 315–382.

86. **Andreasen FM, Vestergaard Pedersen B.** Prognosis of luxated permanent teeth – the development of pulp necrosis. *Endod Dent Traumatol* 1985; **1**: 207–220.

87. **Andreasen FM.** Pulpal healing after luxation injuries and root fracture in the permanent dentition. Thesis, Copenhagen University, 1995. ISBN 87-985538-0-1.

SUBLUXATION

88. **Andreasen FM, Andreasen JO.** Luxation Injuries. In: Andreasen JO, Andreasen FM eds. *Textbook and Color Atlas of Traumatic Injuries to the Teeth*, 3rd edn. Copenhagen: Munksgaard, 1993: 315–382.

89. **Andreasen FM, Vestergaard Pedersen B.** Prognosis of luxated permanent teeth – the development of pulp necrosis. *Endod Dent Traumatol.* 1985; **1**: 207–220.

90. **Andreasen FM.** Pulpal healing after luxation injuries and root fracture in the permanent dentition. Thesis, Copenhagen University, 1995. ISBN 87-985537-0-1.

EXTRUSIVE LUXATION

91. **Andreasen FM, Andreasen JO.** Luxation injuries. In: Andreasen JO, Andreasen FM eds. *Textbook and Color Atlas of Traumatic Injuries to the Teeth*, 3rd edn. Copenhagen: Munksgaard, 1993: 315–378.

92. **Andreasen FM, Vestergaard Pedersen B.** Prognosis of luxated permanent teeth – development of pulp necrosis. *Endod Dent Traumatol* 1985; **1**: 207–220.

93. **Andreasen FM, Yu Z, Thomsen BL.** The relationship between pulpal dimensions and the development of pulp necrosis after luxation injuries in the permanent dentition. *Endod Dent Traumatol* 1986; **2**: 90–98.

94. **Andreasen FM.** Transient apical breakdown and its relation to color and sensibility changes after luxation injuries to teeth. *Endod Dent Traumatol* 1986; **2**: 9–19.

95. **Andreasen FM, Yu Z, Thomsen BL, Anderson PK.** Occurrence of pulp canal obliteration after luxation in the permanent dentition. *Endod Dent Traumatol* 1987; **23**: 103–115.

96. **Oikarinen K, Grundlach KKH, Pfelfer G.** Late complications of luxation injuries to teeth. *Endod Dent Traumatol* 1987; **3**: 296–303.

97. **Rock WP, Grundy MC.** The effect of luxation and subluxation upon the prognosis of traumatized incisor teeth. *Endod Dent Traumatol* 1981; **9**: 224–230.

98. **Stålhane I, Hedegård B.** Traumatized permanent teeth in children aged 7–15 years. Part II. *Swed Dent J* 1975; **68**: 157–169.

99. **Eklund G, Stålhane I, Hedegård B.** A study of traumatized permanent teeth In children aged 7–15 years. Part III. A complications of subluxated and luxated teeth. *Swed Dent J* 1976; **69**: 179–189.

LATERAL LUXATION

100. **Andreasen FM, Andreasen JO.** Luxation injuries. In: Andreasen JO, Andreasen FM eds. *Textbook and Color Atlas of Traumatic Injuries to the Teeth*, 3rd edn. Copenhagen: Munksgaard, 1993: 315–382.

101. **Andreasen FM, Vestergaard Pedersen B.** Prognosis of luxated permanent teeth – the development of pulp necrosis. *Endod Dent Traumatol* 1985; **1**: 207–220.

102. **Andreasen FM.** Pulpal healing after luxation injuries and root fracture in the permanent dentition. Thesis, Copenhagen University, 1995. ISBN 87-985537-0-1.

INTRUSIVE LUXATION

103. **Andreasen FM, Andreasen JO.** Luxation injuries. In: Andreasen JO, Andreasen FM eds. *Textbook and Color Atlas of Traumatic Injuries to the Teeth*, 3rd edn. Copenhagen: Munksgaard, 1993: 315–382.

104. **Andreasen FM.** Pulpal healing after luxation injuries and root fracture in the permanent dentition. Thesis, Copenhagen University, 1995. ISBN 87-985537-0-1.

105. **Andreasen FM, Vestrgaard Pedersen B.** Prognosis of luxated permanent teeth – the development of pulp necrosis. *Endod Dent Traumatol* 1985; **1**: 207–220.

106. **Andreasen FM, Yu z Thomsen BL.** The relationship between pulpal dimensions and the development of pulp necrosis after luxation injuries in the permanent dentition. *Endod Dent Traumatol* 1986; **2**: 90–98.

107. **Ebeleseder KA, Santler G, Glockner K, Hulla H, Pertl C, Quenhenberger F.** An analysis of 58 traumatically intruded and surgically extruded permanent teeth. *Endod Dent Traumatol.* 2000; **16**: 34–39.

108. **Kinirons MJ, Sutcliffe J.** Traumatically intruded permanent incisors: a study of treatment and outcome. *Br Dent J* 1991; **170**: 144–146.

109. **Andreasen JO, Andreasen FM.** Intrusion of permanent teeth. An analysis of 115 teeth, 2003. Study in progress.

AVULSION

110. **Andreasen JO, Andreasen FM.** Avulsions. In: Andreasen JO, Andreasen FM eds. *Textbook and Color Atlas of Traumatic Injuries to the Teeth*, 3rd edn. Copenhagen: Munksgaard, 1993: 383–420.

111. **Andreasen JO.** Replantation of avulsed teeth. In: Andreasen JO, Andreasen FM eds. *Textbook and Color Atlas of Traumatic Injuries to the Teeth*, 3rd edn. Copenhagen: Munksgaard, 1993: 57–97.

112. **Andreasen JO, Borum M, Jacobsen HL, Andreasen FM.** Replantation of 400 traumatically avulsed permanent incisors. I. Diagnosis of healing complications. *Endod Dent Traumatol* 1995; **11**: 51–58.

113. **Andreasen JO, Borum M, Jacobsen HL, Andreasen FM.** Replantation of 400 avulsed permanent incisors. II. Factors

related to pulp healing. *Endod Dent Traumatol* 1995; **11**: 59–68.

114. **Andreasen JO, Borum M, Jacobsen HL, Andreasen FM.** Replantation of 400 avulsed permanent incisors. III. Factors related to root growth after replantation. *Endod Dent Traumatol* 1995; **11**: 69–75.

115. **Andreasen JO, Borum M, Jacobsen HL, Andreasen FM.** Replantation of 400 avulsed permanent incisors. IV. Factors related to periodontal ligament healing. *Endod Dent Traumatol* 1995; **11**: 76–89.

116. **Andreasen JO, Borum M, Andreasen FM.** Progression of root resorption after replantation of 400 avulsed human incisors. In: Davidovitch Z ed. *The Biological Mechanisms of Tooth Eruption, Resorption and Replacement by Implants.* Boston, MA: Harvard Society for the Advancement of Orthodontics, 1994: 577–582.

117. **Andreasen JO.** Periodontal healing after repolantation of traumatically avulsed human teeth. Assessment by mobility testing and radiography. *Acta Odontol Scand* 1975; **33**: 325–335.

118. **Cvek M, Granath LE, Hollender L.** Treatment of non-vital permanent incisors with calcium hydroxide. III. Variation of occurrence of ankylosis of reimplanted teeth with duration of extra-alveolar period and storage enviroment. *Odont Revy* 1974; **25**: 43–56.

119. **American Association of Endodontists.** Treatment of the avulsed permanent tooth. Recommended Guidelines of the American Association of Endodontists, 1995.

120. **Barrett EJ, Kenny DJ.** Avulsed permanent teeth: a review of the literature and treament guidelines. *Endod Dent Traumatol* 1997; **13**: 153–163.

121. **Barrett EJ, Kenny DJ.** Survival of avulsed permanent maxillary incisors in children following delayed replantation. *Endod Dent Traumatol* 1997; **13**: 269–275.

122. **Boyd DH, Kinirons MJ, Gregg TA.** A prospective study of factors effecting survival of replanted permanent incisors in children. *Int J Paediatric Dent* 2000; **10**: 200–205.

123. **Kinirons MJ, Gregg TA, Welbury RR, Cole BO.** Variations in the presenting and treatment features in reimplantated permanent incisors in children and their effect on the prevalence of root resorption. *Br Dent J* 200; **189**: 263–266.

124. **Kinirons MJ, Boyd DH, Gregg TA.** Inflammatory and replacement resorption in reimplanted permanent incisors teeth: a study of the characteristics of 84 teeth. *Endod Dent Traumatol* 1999; **15**: 269–272.

125. **Mackie IC, Worthington HV.** An investigation of replantation of traumatically avulsed permanent incisor teeth. *Br Dent J* 1992; **172**: 17–20.

126. **Schatz JP, Hausherr C, Joho JP.** A retrospective clinical and radiologic study of teeth re-implanted following traumatic avulsion. *Endod Dent Traumatol* 1995; 11: 235–239.

127. **Trope M, Friedman S.** Periodontal healing of replanted dog teeth stored in Viaspan, milk and Hank's balanced salt solution. *Endod Dent* 1992; **8**: 183–188.

128. **Coccia CT.** A clinical investigation of root resorption rates in reimplanted young permanent incisors: a five-year study. *J Endod* 1980; **6**: 413–420.

129. **Kling M, Cvek M, Mejare I.** Rate and predictability of pulp revascularization in therapeuticically reimplanted permanent incisors. *Endod Dent Traumatol* 1986; **2**: 83–89.

130. **Andersson L, Blomlöf L, Lindskog S, Feiglin B, Hammerström L.** Tooth ankylosis. Clinical, radiographic and histological assessments. *Int J Oral Surg* 1984; **13**: 423–431.

131. **Kawanami M, Andreasen JO, Borum MK, Schou S, Hjørting-Hansen E, Kato H.** Infraposition of ankylosed permanent maxillary incisors after replantation related to age and sex. *Endod Dent Traumatol* 1999; **15**: 50–56.

INJURIES TO THE PRIMARY DENTITION

132. **Andreasen JO.** Injuries to developing teeth. In: Andreasen JO, Andreasen FM eds. *Textbook and Color Atlas of Traumatic Injuries to the Teeth*, 3rd edn. Copenhagen: Munksgaard, 1993: 459–491.

133. **Borum MK, Andreasen JO.** Sequelae of trauma to primary mixillary incisors. I. Complications in the primary dentition. *Endod Dent Traumatol* 1998; **14**: 31–44.

134. **Andreasen JO, Sundström B, Ravn JJ.** The effect of traumatic injuries to primary teeth on their permanent successors. I. A clinical and histologic study of 117 injured permanent teeth. *Scand J Dent Res* 1971; **79**: 219–283.

135. **Andreasen JO, Ravn JJ.** The effect of traumatic injuries to primary teeth on their permanent successors. II. A clinical and radiographic follow-up study of 213 injured teeth. *Scand J Dent Res* 1971; **79**: 284–294.

136. **Andreasen JO, Ravn JJ.** Enamel changes in permanent teeth after trauma of their primary predecessors. *Scand J Dent Res* 1973; **81**: 203–209.

137. **Selliseth N-E.** The significance of traumatised primary incisors on the development and eruption of permanent teeth. *Eur Orthodont Dent Soc* 1970; **46**: 443–459.

138. **Ben Bassat Y, Brin I, Fuks A, Zilberman Y.** Effect of trauma to the primary incisors on permanent successors in different developmental stages. *Pediatr Dent* 1985; **7**: 37–40.

139. **Zilberman Y, Ben Bassat Y, Lustmann J.** Effect of trauma to primary incisors on root development to their permanent successors. *Pediatr Dent* 1986; **8**: 289–293.

140. **von Arx T.** Traumatologie im Milchgebiss (I). Klinische und therapeutische Aspekte. *Schweiz Monatsschr Zahnmed* 1990; **100**: 1195–1204.

141. **von Arx T.** Traumatologie im Milchgebiss (II). Langzeitergebnisse sowie Auswirkungen auf das Milchgebiss und die bleibende Dentition. *Schwiz Monatsschr Zahnmed* 1991; **101**: 57–68.

SPLINTING

142. **Andreasen FM, Andreasen JO.** Luxation injuries. In: Andreasen JO, Andreasen FM eds. *Textbook and Color Atlas of Traumatic Injuries to the Teeth*, 3rd edn. Copenhagen: Munksgaard, 1993: 315–382.

143. **Mandel U, Viidik A.** Effect of splinting on the mechanical and histological properties of the healing periodontal ligament in the vervet monkey (*Cercopithecus aethiops*). *Arch Oral Biol* 1989; **34**: 209–217.

144. **Andreasen JO.** The effect of splinting upon periodontal and pulpal healing after replantation of permanent incisors in monkeys. *Acta Odontal Scand* 1975; **33**: 313–323.

145. **Kristerson L, Andreasen JO.** The effect of splinting upon periodontal and pulpal healing after autotransplantation of mature and immature permanent incisors in monkeys. *Int J Oral Surg* 1983; **12**: 239–249.

146. **Andreasen JO.** Experimental dental traumatology: development of a model for external root resorption. *Endod Dent Traumatol* 1987; **3**: 260–287.

147. **Oikarinen K.** Functional fixation for traumatically luxated teeth. *Endod Dent Traumatol* 1987; **3**: 224–228.

148. **Oikarinen K.** Comparison of the flexibility of various splinting methods for tooth fixation. *J Oral Maxillofac Surg* 1988; **17**: 225–227.

149. **Oikarinen K.** Tooth splinting: a review of the literature and consideration of the versatility of a wire-composite splint. *Endod Dent Traumatol* 1990; **6**: 237–250.

150. **Oikarinen K, Andreasen JO, Andreasen FM.** Rigidity of various fixation methods used as dental splints. *Endod Dent Traumatol* 1992; **8**: 113–119.

ENDODONTIC IMPLICATIONS OF DENTAL TRAUMA

151. **Cvek M.** Endodontic management of traumatized teeth. In: Andreasen JO, Andreasen FM eds. *Textbook and Color Atlas of Traumatic Injuries to the Teeth*, 3rd edn. Copenhagen: Munksgaard, 1993: 517–585.

152. **Andersen M, Lund A, Andreasen JO, Andreasen FM.** In vitro solidity of human pulp tissue in calcium hydroxite and sodium hypochlorite. *Endod Dent Traumatol* 1992; **8**: 104–108.

153. **Andreasen JO, Farik B, Munksgaard EC.** Long-term calcium hydroxide as a root canal dressing may increase risk of root fracture. *Dent Traumatol* 2002; **18**: 134–137.

154. **Cvek M.** Prognosis of luxated non-vital maxillary incisors treated with calcium hydroxite and filled with gutta-percha. *Endod Dent Traumatol* 1992; **8**: 45–55.

155. **Torabinejad M, Watson TF, Pitt Ford TR.** The sealing ability of a mineral trioxide aggregate as a retrograde root filling material. *J Endodon* 1993; **19**: 591–595.

156. **Torabinejad M, Hong CU, Ptt Ford TR.** Physical and chemical properties of a new root end filling material. *J Endodon* 1995; **21**: 349–353.

157. **Pitt Ford TR, Torabinejad M, Abedi HR, Bakland LK, Kariyawasam SP.** Mineral trioxide aggregate as a pulp capping material. *J Am Dent Ass* 1996; **127**: 1491–1494.

158. **Torabinejad M, Chivian N.** Clinical applications of mineral trioxide aggregate. *J Endod* 1999; **25**: 197–205.

159. **Faraco IM Jr, Holland R.** Response of the pulp of dogs to capping with mineral trioxide aggregate or a calcium hydroxide cement. *Dent Traumatol* 2001; **17**: 163–66.

160. **Tziafas D, Pantelidou O, Alvanou A, Belibasakis G, Papadimitriou S.** The dentinogenic effect of mineral trioxide aggregate (MTA) in short-term capping experiments. *Int Endod J* 2002; **35**: 245–254.

161. **Shabahang S, Torabinejad M.** Treatment of teeth with open apices using mineral trioxide aggregate. *Pract Periodont Aesthet Dent* 2000; **12**: 315–320.

162. **Giuliani V, Baccetti T, Pace R, Pagavino G.** The use of MTA in teeth with necrotic pulps and open apices. *Dent Traumatol* 2002; **18**: 217–221.

TOOTH SURVIVAL FOLLOWING VARIOUS TRAUMA ENTITIES IN THE PERMANENT DENTITION

163. **Andreasen JO, Andreasen FM, Robertson A.** Long-term prognosis of 1587 traumatized permanent teeth, 2003. Study in progress.

INFORMATION TO THE PUBLIC ABOUT DENTAL TRAUMA

164. **US Department of Health and Human Services.** Community and other approaches to promote oral health and prevent oral disease. In: *Oral Health in America: A Report of the Surgeon General*. Rockville, MD: US Department of Health and Human Services, National Institute of Dental and Craniofacial Research, National Institutes of Health, 2000: chapter 7.

165. **Tsukiboshi M.** *If You Know It, You Can Save the Tooth on Trauma*. Tokyo: Quintessence Publishing, 1996.

166. **Andreasen FM.** *O. Clast & the Bros. Blast*. Fribourg: Mediglobe, 1988.

167. Recommendations on selected interventions to prevent dental caries, oral and pharyngeal cancers, and sports-related craniofacial injuries. *Am J Prev Med* 2002; **23**: 16–20.

168. **Traumatismo Dental Infantil**. Información práctica y primeros auxilios. Servicio Traumatología Dental Infantil Universidad de Valparaíso, Chile 2002. http://www.uv.cl/stdi/comunidad/avulsion.htm

169. **Atlantic Amateur Hockey Association.** Mouth Guards; Understanding the Facts, 2002. http://www.sportsdds.com/hockey1.htm

170. **International Academy for Sports Dentistry.** Trauma Card, 2002. http://www.sportsdentistry-iads.org/trauma.htm

171. **American Association of Endodontists.** Your Guide to Traumatic Dental Injuries, 2002. http://www.aae.org/traumsum.html

172. **American Academy of Pediatric Dentistry.** Emergency Care, 2002. http://www.aapd.org/publications/brochures/ecare.asp

173. **ADA Public Service Announcements (PSAs).** *Soccer Moms: Mouth Guards*, 2002. http://www.ada.org/public/media/psa/psa-mouthguards.html

PREVENTION OF TRAUMATIC DENTAL AND MAXILLO-FACIAL INJURIES

174. **Stuart MJ, Smith AM, Malo-Ortiguera SA, Fischer TL, Larson DR**. A comparison of facial protection and the incidence of head, neck, and facial injuries in Junior A hockey players. A function of individual playing time. *Am J Sports Med* 2002; **30**: 39–44.

175. **Yamada T, Sawaki Y, Tomida S, Tohnai I, Ueda M.** Oral injury and mouthguard usage by athletes in Japan. *Endod Dent Traumatol* 1998; **14**: 84–87.

176. **Kvittem B, Hardie NA, Roettger M, Conry J.** Incidence of orofacial injuries in high school sports. *J Public Health Dent* 1998; **58**: 288–293.

177. **Castaldi CL.** Mouth guards in contact sports. *J Connecticut State Dent Assoc* 1974; **48**: 233–241.

178. **Hayrinen-Immonen R, Sane J, Perkki K, Malmstrom M.** A six-year follow-up study of sports-related dental injuries in children and adolescents. *Endod Dent Traumatol* 1990; **6**: 208–212.

179. **Scheer, B.** Prevention of dental and oral injuries. In: Andreasen JO, Andreasen FM eds. *Textbook and Color Atlas of Traumatic Injuries to the Teeth*, 3rd edn. Copenhagen: Munksgaard, 1994: 719–735.

180. **Johnston T, Messer LB.** An in vitro study of the efficacy of mouthguard protection for dentoalveolar injuries in deciduous and mixed dentitions. *Endod Dent Traumatol* 1996; **12**: 277–285.

181. **Hoffmann J, Alfter G, Rudolph NK, Goz G.** Experimental comparative study of various mouthguards. *Endod Dent Traumatol* 1999; **15**: 157–163.

182. **McNutt T, Shannon SW, Wright JT, Feistein RA.** Oral trauma in adolescent athletes: a study of mouth guards. *Pediatric Dentistry* 1989; **11**: 205–213.

183. **Nysether S.** Dental injuries among Norwegian soccer players. *Community Dent Oral Epidemiol* 1987; **15**: 141–143.

184. **Oikarinen KS, Salonen MA.** Introduction to four custom-made mouth protectors constructed of single and double layers for activists in contact sports. *Endod Dent Traumatol* 1993; **9**: 19–24.

185. **Truman BI, Gooch BF, Sulemana I, Gift HC, Horowitz AM, Evans CA, et al.** Reviews of evidence on interventions to prevent dental caries, oral and pharyngeal cancers, and sports-related craniofacial injuries. *Am J Prev Med* 2002; **23**: 21–54.

186. **Sane J.** Comparison of maxillofacial and dental injuries in four contact team sports: American football, bandy, basketball, and handball. *Am J Sports Med* 1988; **16**: 647–651.

187. **Maestrello-de Moya MG, Primosch RE.** Orofacial trauma and mouth-protector wear among high school varsity basketball players. *ASDC J Dent Child* 1989; **56**: 36–39.

188. **Labella CR, Smith BW, Sigurdsson A.** Effect of mouthguards on dental injuries and concussions in college basketball. *Med Sci Sports Exerc* 2002; **34**: 41–44.

189. **de Cardenas SO**. Mouth protectors during the 1st World Amateur Boxing Championship. *Rev Cubana Estomatol* 1975; **12**: 49–66.

190. **Vulcan AP, Cameron MH, Watson WL.** Mandatory bicycle helmet use: experience in Victoria, Australia. *World J Surg* 1992; **16**: 389–397.

191. **Acton CH, Nixon JW, Clark RC.** Bicycle riding and oral/maxillofacial trauma in young children. *Med J Aust* 1996; **165**: 249–251.

192. **Linn S, Smith D, Sheps S.** Epidemiology of bicycle injury, head injury and helmet use among children in British Colombia: a five year descriptive study. Canadian hospitals injury reporting and prevention program (CHIRPP). *Inj Prev* 1998; **4**: 122–125.

193. **Thompson DC, Nunn MF, Thompson RS, Rivara FP.** Effectiveness of bicycle safety helmets in preventing serious facial injury. *J Amer Med Ass* 1997; **276**: 1774–1775.

194. **Kelly P, Sanson T, Strange G, Orsay E.** A prospective study of the impact of helmet usage on motorcycle trauma. *Ann Emerg Med* 1991; **20**: 852–856.

195. **Bachulis BL, Sanster W, Gorrell GW, et al.** Patterns of injury in helmet and nonhelmet motorcyclists. *Am J Surg* 1988; **155**: 708–711.

196. **Reath DB, Kirby J, Lynch M, Maull KI.** Patterns of maxillofacial injuries in restrained and unrestrained motor vehicle crash victims. *J Trauma* 1989; **29**: 806–809.

Index